Having Sex, Wanting Intimacy

HAVING SEX, WANTING INTIMACY

Why Women Settle for One-Sided Relationships

JILL P. WEBER

ROWMAN & LITTLEFIELD PUBLISHERS, INC.
Lanham • Boulder • New York • Toronto • Plymouth, UK

Published by Rowman & Littlefield Publishers, Inc.
A wholly owned subsidiary of
The Rowman & Littlefield Publishing Group, Inc.
4501 Forbes Boulevard, Suite 200, Lanham, Maryland 20706
www.rowman.com

10 Thornbury Road, Plymouth PL6 7PP, United Kingdom

British Library Cataloguing in Publication Information Available

Library of Congress Cataloging-in-Publication Data

Weber, Jill P., 1973–
Having sex, wanting intimacy : why women settle for one-sided relationships / Jill P. Weber.
p. cm
Includes bibliographical references and index.
ISBN 978-1-4422-2020-1 (pbk. : alk. paper) — ISBN 978-1-4422-2021-8 (electronic)
1. Interpersonal relations. 2. Women—Sexual behavior. I. Title.
HM1106.W434 2013
306.7082—dc23

2012032390

∞™ The paper used in this publication meets the minimum requirements of American National Standard for Information Sciences—Permanence of Paper for Printed Library Materials, ANSI/NISO Z39.48-1992.

Printed in the United States of America

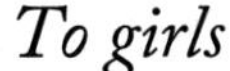

To girls

CONTENTS

PREFACE

Sextimacy is the effort to find emotional intimacy through sex. It may seem to offer a woman a shortcut to happiness at first, but when it becomes habitual, the result is frustration and disappointment.

A common step in this process is the adoption by some women of the conventional male strategy, even a male point of view, for dating. Women who step in this direction may feel as if they are taking control of their romantic lives, and then with time, this feeling passes, to be replaced by a sharp sense of emotional isolation.

I coined the word *sextimacy* to facilitate communication in therapy. "Promiscuous," "wild," "fast," the generalization "hooking up," and similar words are often used in a judgmental way that impedes objective analysis. It's not that these words don't have uses, but as labels they amplify the discomfort that women may feel about their sexuality and derail productive introspection. My experience with patients has shown me, firsthand, the clarity that an uninhibited discussion of sextimacy can bring to adolescent girls and young and middle-aged women. Clarity, perhaps above all, helps women become attentive to their own needs.

With this book, I hope that the word *sextimacy* will help identify a concern that, outside of the privacy of psychotherapy offices, does not get the public attention it deserves. It also helps parents who desperately want to protect their daughters from all that can go wrong in the process of experimenting with romance. Those I deal with are often visibly relieved to have sextimacy explained. It gives parents and their daughters a road map that helps them communicate in productive ways. The urge to give in to panic dissipates, and they often become significantly closer to their daughters as a result.

Sextimacy occurs on a spectrum. Many intuitively sense the hazard and proceed with caution. Some hope a casual liaison will be the beginning of a journey that will lead to emotional intimacy and commitment. In other cases, emotional intimacy is not the woman's expressed initial goal. For others still, sextimacy may become their only avenue for forging romantic relationships with men. What seems to them to be a path to emotional intimacy leads instead to a cul-de-sac, circling and circling in a disappointing, sometimes heartbreaking cycle. In the last instance, women explain the disappointments to themselves with self-blame and then, paradoxically, try to repair their negative feelings with another sextimacy encounter and then another. And in all of these cases, sextimacy may occur in the proverbial one-night stand or, more perversely and more typically, occur in a series of emotionally sterile sexual encounters with the same man.

There is an ongoing cultural media-promoted fantasy about sex and intimacy that purports by some magic of happenstance that two people will careen together and, presto, true love will reign. It is a formula used for many books and movies. The simplicity of the story is appealing. But life and more serious fiction are more complicated than that.

These and other cultural, as well as family, influences set up some girls to become adults who settle for one-sided relationships where their needs are not being met. Many girls are socialized to subordinate their feelings. They are schooled to be "nice" at all times, however they might actually feel, and to go along to get along. Unfortunately, these messages may ultimately become quite self-destructive. Women may suppress their deep desire to be fully known and adopt a belief that men can't handle their truth. These women typically hold out hope that somehow, if they suppress enough, their relationships will eventually deliver what they desire—emotional intimacy. They won't.

Having Sex, Wanting Intimacy is about helping women discover what it is that drives their happiness in romantic relationships, and it is about women who are trapped by the need to perpetually sacrifice in order to maintain their connections with men.

Many women grow up fully equipped to form fulfilling, emotionally intimate relationships with men. But many don't. Happily, those who don't can learn to alter their behavior in ways that will improve their prospects for love. As women no longer allow themselves to settle for the dregs, some men are challenged to look at their own character. If this process means that a woman leaves some men behind, the comfort is in knowing that all will be better for it.

After completing this book, I learned I was pregnant with a baby girl. Although a dream come true, I find myself daunted, overwhelmed by the emotional weight of my own girl and her future. How will my husband and I even begin to spar with and counter the many unavoidable, bogus messages about femininity that abound? I find a measure of confidence by remembering that which has been protective for me and for the women and girls I have treated professionally and have known personally. And this is the power of candid, accepting relationships with others—between mothers and daughters, fathers and daughters, sisters, friends, colleagues, teachers, therapists, and coaches.

When a woman or a girl finds herself in the presence of another who is truly open to her experience, without judgment or blocks to intimacy, she is drawn closer to her authentic self. By steadfastly staying in tune with herself, it becomes easier to separate her own desires from those of others and from the ever-moving judgment of culture.

The women I see in my practice inspire. Their willingness to confront their disappointments is an ongoing demonstration of what women can accomplish for themselves. In each case described, details of individual stories have been significantly altered so as to preserve confidential identity. In addition, identity is concealed by only using cases that reflect compilations of recurring themes.

1

THE QUICK FIX

Sextimacy Defined

While writing this book, I attended a bachelorette party for a thirty-something bride-to-be in New York City. On a whim, we entered Hogs and Heifers, a well-known bar in Manhattan devoted to providing bachelorettes with a last few moments of entertainment before they wed. As soon as you enter this bar, it is clear the women are in charge—hopped up on adrenaline and Pabst Blue Ribbon, wearing tight-fitting tank tops and stilettoes, hurling their bras onto the bar as they groove to music from the jukebox. One of the bartenders—beautiful, early twenties—dances on top of the bar in a bikini, while using a megaphone to shout insults at the men who enter: "Get out of here, punk," "Is that your ass or your face?," or sounding a siren while cheering into a megaphone, "Ladies, we got ourselves a hot one here . . . finally." The women in the bar grind with one another on the dance floor as guys beg for a dance, only to be aggressively pushed away unless they are deemed, by the standards of the room, hot and gorgeous.

This shameless spectacle of women acting nothing like the female stereotypes of sweet and nice is alluring and seductive. The control they exude and their take-charge attitude is infectious, so much more powerful than a passive lady-in-waiting. And, yet, as the siren sounded one more time, I recognized this as a fantasy world and realized that I know these young women. Perhaps I know a side they only show a privileged few, but I do know them—intimately. I know that under this tough exterior is vulnerability, along with a desire to feel intimately and deeply connected with the men in their lives. I also know that many women choose a life of what I call "sextimacy"—pursuing sex to gain emotional intimacy—out of feeling overwhelmed and crippled by the many sexual dilemmas that are present for women in our culture. I know they feel forced into a male model of dating that barters sex for an emotional connection. I also know they are caught between believing they should be self-sufficient without a man, all the while craving true intimacy.

As a result of these dilemmas, and left with the understandable perception that there are no viable options, some women have found a way to level the playing field: sextimacy. For a surprising number of women, sextimacy is the primary means for forging relationships with men. Many young women are embarrassed to openly admit to themselves or to other women that a "real" relationship is what they desire. These women have come to believe that wanting emotional intimacy with someone with whom they also have sex is weak and needy, a sort of sappy female stereotype. They live out a young adult life of publicly shouting from a megaphone that they "Don't care about feelings and love" or they "Don't have time for relationships," while privately they fantasize about one of their hookups eventually leading to the end of the rainbow, where they may finally become a "we."

In reality, sextimacy is no choice at all; invariably the woman is left with striking disappointment because it never delivers what she deeply desires—a real relationship. In my practice as a clinical psychologist, I often talk with women who are fed up with sextimacy and bravely admit that all they really want is to have a meaningful, mutual connection with someone whom they adore and who adores them in return. The problem these women face is that, within the present culture of dating and hooking up, they do not know how to form lasting, meaningful, truly intimate relationships with men. One such example is Julia.

Julia, a twenty-two-year-old single law-school student, is getting ready for a night out with friends. As she picks out her outfit and does her hair, she notices she feels hopeful and optimistic, a contrast from the depressed feelings she felt earlier in the day. She is excited by the thought that tonight she might meet Mr. Right. As she dresses to get ready, she imagines how the evening will transpire. Perhaps he will be at the end of the bar, appearing aloof and mysterious. She will be with her friends and will notice him noticing her. There will be side-glances, and she will see that he is attractive. Eventually, he will approach, and an instant connection will be made; she will see immediate interest and engagement in his eyes. Their initial meeting will be followed by an abundance of hand holding, touching, and exchanging information about themselves. They will find all sorts of commonalities in their personalities and uncanny coincidences from their backgrounds. By the next day, they will already have a date in place to meet again, and they will become inseparable. In Julia's mind, it will feel easy and blissful, almost like a story in a movie or a love song. The fantasy is compelling and eases her feelings of loneliness and emptiness.

By the time she goes out that evening, she is well primed to meet her life partner, and, in fact, she meets a guy that evening. They exchange personal information and discover common interests. Julia greatly enjoys getting to know this shiny new man, and his instant interest in and attraction to her feels wonderful. His level of engagement makes her feel special and worthy. Their chemistry is smoking, and it feels natural for Julia to cap off the evening with sex. However, once sexual contact begins to progress, she feels alone and unsure of herself. By the time it is over, Julia feels downright empty and entirely regrets the sexual event. The lifelong-partner-enduring-connection-read-your-thoughts-and-attend-to-your-every-need part of her fantasy does not happen. By 8:00 a.m. Sunday morning, the new guy is gone; he does not even suggest breakfast. Julia is left feeling emptier and more depressed than ever.

Sextimacy is a combination of the words *sex* and *intimacy* and refers to the search for emotional closeness through sex, whereby sex or hooking up is used to the exclusion of other methods for developing a connection such as dating, friendship, and shared participation in activities. The frequency of sextimacy experiences varies among women. In some cases, there may be just a few episodes. At the extreme, sextimacy becomes a way of life and the only avenue used to develop relationships with men. Sextimacy often starts in the teenage years and peaks in young adulthood. For some women, it continues throughout young adulthood and, for others, recurs in the context of marriage through extramarital affairs.

This book is written to help those who want the ability to self-correct as they assess their sextimacy experiences, and, most particularly, it is written for those who struggle to develop the ability to escape from a sextimacy trap. It takes work and self-analysis, but relief is available. As women develop healthier relationships with themselves, they become better equipped to forge authentic and mutually beneficial relationships with men. The strategies in this book will help women make conscious choices about when and with whom to have sex/hook up and how to keep their best interest in mind when making such choices.

As a clinical psychologist, I see teenagers, young women, and married women in my practice who suffer from sextimacy. Although these women tell me they are looking for long-term acceptance and commitment from the men in their lives, their actions tell a different story. Sextimacy is a self-defeating cycle. The sex never ultimately delivers what women are so longing for: a nurturing, mutually fulfilling relationship that provides both sexual and emotional intimacy. After a sextimacy event, many women may feel worse and emptier than before. The cycle continues with feelings of worthlessness giving rise to yet another sextimacy event.

When sextimacy occurs for teenagers, the toll is cumulative and progressive. As the adolescent moves through each stage of development, it becomes more difficult to cultivate a romantic connection without the early introduction of sex. As the teenage years pass and romantic connections are forged through hastened sex, the young adult misses opportunities to learn how to develop sustained and mutually fulfilling connections with men. If this pattern continues into the early twenties, the woman is left feeling entirely ill-equipped to manage the complexities of a long-term committed relationship. Developing a romantic relationship without the early introduction of sex comes to feel awkward for the woman because she has not developed a sense of her worth outside of a sexual context.

Women who repeatedly engage in sextimacy experience emotional and relational difficulties. At the heart of these trials is a lack of understanding and acceptance of themselves. Adolescent girls and adult women in a pattern of sextimacy feel painfully self-conscious about their bodies, their mood is often down or depressed, and they engage in repetitive negative thinking. They feel uncomfortable with intimacy, which makes it hard for them to both find a committed partner and to be a committed partner. They feel alone and unfulfilled. They have difficulty understanding their emotional world, which makes it challenging for them to communicate effectively so they can get their needs met by the men in their lives. These roadblocks have them turn once again to sex as a tool to attain momentary relief from low self-esteem and hopelessness. Chronic sextimacy leaves a woman with little opportunity to develop the emotional and relational skills she needs in order to form a meaningful relationship. And, without these skills, she becomes more vulnerable to repeated sextimacy events.

Because sextimacy circumvents the hard work of relationship development, women who have not been exposed to attentive relationships in childhood are more at risk for a sextimacy dynamic to permeate their adult romantic relationships. Biological and environmental factors along with caregiver responses (as outlined in chapter 3) leave some girls vulnerable to emotional neglect. Common family dynamics that may contribute to sextimacy for a young woman include parents with highly conflicted marriages, parental abandonment, parents who have other children with serious medical or psychological issues, parents who relocate or move a great deal, and parents who have their own psychological issues. Frequently, sextimacy creeps into a young woman's life at no fault of a caregiver; the culture at large and peer group influence alone can account for its development (as outlined in chapter 2).

In general, these factors condition many women to expect and tolerate one-directional relationships—where their needs go unmet or are sacrificed for the needs of others. Below are examples of women's experiences with sextimacy in the context of marriage, the teen years, and young adulthood.

SEXTIMACY WITHIN MARRIAGE

When a marriage is in trouble, there are various ways that couples act out their conflicts, and sexual affairs represent one of these ways. For some women affairs represent returning to an old coping style, a way to regain some sense of self-validation amidst an emotional storm. When a woman's sexual coming-of-age involved using sextimacy as a way to pursue emotional closeness with men, it is easy to revert.

Monica, thirty-five years old and married, was shocked when she found herself suddenly wrapped up in an intense affair with a male coworker. She entered psychotherapy treatment overwhelmed by emotion; she felt guilty and confused by her feelings, yet compelled to see this man. She was distressed that she had allowed herself to fall into an affair and was painfully self-critical. As we explored Monica's past, we discovered that her introduction to the sexual world was through sextimacy. She reported that throughout her childhood, her family moved every year for professional reasons. She was always the new girl in school and felt excluded and alone in this role. She learned by eighth grade that making herself sexually available to her teenage male counterparts enabled her to have a degree of acceptance. She recalled instances where she might feel down at not being invited to a classmate's party and then thrilled when a guy would call her, out of the blue, for a late evening rendezvous. The day after a hookup, Monica would pass the boy in the hallway at school, and although he would not speak to her, she felt special knowing that he had wanted her the night before.

There were several insidious side effects to this mode of developing peer acceptance. For one, the feeling of being liked wore off quickly, which left Monica perpetually in search of her next quick fix. Between hookups, Monica felt empty and ashamed. She had trouble feeling good about what she "had to do" to keep men in her life. Finally, as Monica's high school years went by, so too did the opportunities to build her self-esteem and to learn the skills necessary to forge mutually fulfilling relationships with men.

By the time she entered college, she was socially anxious around men who wanted to date and get to know her. Each time she went on a date or spent time one-on-one with a man in a context that did not involve sexual contact, she felt self-conscious and awkward. Monica would become so anxious that she would impulsively make the relationship sexual as soon as possible. This coping mechanism offered Monica a short reprieve, as the men involved were more than willing to accommodate. Nonetheless, once the encounter was over, she was left to feel even more self-conscious and internally defeated. She believed ultimate acceptance and a genuine connection with a man were permanently out of her reach.

This kind of dating, quickly short-circuiting to sex, eventually paid off, and Monica committed to a man and married. However, the hurry-up process did not require her husband to actually get to know more than one dimension of her. In order for this relationship to work, she became a chameleon, taking on the identity of her husband. Monica embraced the same interests and likes as her husband. He enjoyed basketball. She made sure to surprise him with tickets regularly. He liked steak. She liked steak. He wanted to spend more time with his family. She stopped seeing her own. After five years of marriage, Monica recognized that her husband did not know her because she never revealed her true self.

As a consequence of not feeling known and genuinely valued by her husband, Monica reverted to her old coping strategy and became easily drawn into an affair with a coworker. The cycle from her past repeated; she felt a temporary self-esteem surge, followed by prolonged feelings of guilt and shame, which she managed by negative self-appraisals: "I am an awful person . . . I am a horrible wife . . . No one will ever like me for who I am . . . I am weak . . . How could anyone want to be with me?" These painfully harsh judgments led to a depleted self, which then fueled an even stronger need for instant validation by way of another round of sextimacy.

THE REPEATED HOOKUP

Another context in which sextimacy is used as a tool for developing a relationship with a man is through repeatedly hooking up with the same person. "Hooking up" refers to any type of sexual behavior, including intercourse but also may be limited to oral sex or making out. Although the couple may continue this for weeks, months, and even years, the relationship does not progress on any level. This is a virulent strain of sextimacy because it can be excruciatingly difficult for a woman to extricate herself from this dynamic. The woman engaging in the repeated hookup is perpetually caught in a tug-of-war: one moment no longer wanting to be involved with the person, and the next moment wanting nothing more than to be intimate with this same person. For some women it can be like jumping up and down on a trampoline, feeling high at times and falling lower than low at others.

This sextimacy dynamic is pernicious because it is intermittently reinforced. As we know, behaviors reoccur when they are reinforced. A dog that gets a treat when it sits will learn to sit on command. A more complicated variant of this same phenomenon is intermittent reinforcement, which occurs when something is reinforced some of the time and not at other times. Research has shown that intermittent reinforcement is the most powerful way to increase behavior recurrence. If going to the same fishing spot sometimes yields a catch, and at other times does not, the angler will likely try that spot again and again. Our brains tell us if it happened once, it can happen again. It is easy to deny the possibility that the desired event will either not occur at all or that something worse will.

This is precisely why the repeated hookup continues, sometimes over years—there is always the possibility that it will turn into a real relationship. Perhaps in the late hours, the male involved may even state a desire for a dating relationship or express some kind of jealousy about other men in the woman's life. The woman often experiences this emoting as a sign that there is hope. If she only holds on, this man may be able to deliver not only sex, but also the acceptance, friendship, and companionship for which she longs. She agrees to another late night outing, and not only does he fail to mention anything about wanting to get to know her better, but he also asks her to leave immediately after they have sex. She feels more depleted than ever. In an effort to regain her self-esteem and reclaim her dignity, she is now even more vulnerable to hooking up again with this same person. The next encounter may go well, in that the woman may hear the words she wants to hear, but inevitably the pullback will reoccur, and the cycle will repeat.

Britney was a social and outgoing seventeen-year-old. Although she had many male and female friends and a large social network, she felt left out because she did not have a boyfriend. She wanted to fall in love and share herself fully with someone who would understand and support her. Britney was drawn to Drew, a popular, outgoing friend in her school. Drew was larger than life—funny, extroverted, and extremely attractive. Drew and Britney did not interact at school, but when she got home, he often contacted her online or through text. He tried to get to know her and asked questions that made her feel as though he was interested in more than sex.

After texting, they saw each other at a party the next weekend. They were both drinking when, in the spirit of the moment, they decided to hook up. Britney immediately felt a surge in her self-esteem. She felt bigger than life, just like Drew, and more accepted because he was interested in her. For a few days, she did not hear from him online or at school and told herself that he was probably busy—she should play it cool and not be "needy" or overly "dramatic."

Days turned into weeks and still no real contact. When Britney passed Drew in the hallway at school, he would sort of joke with her and quickly give her a high-five as he passed by. This was not the kind of connection she expected to develop between them. She felt depressed, as if all of her hopes were crashing down. As a matter of fact, she felt worse than before Drew took an interest in her because now she felt he was rejecting her. Soon after Britney felt Drew withdraw his interest, she began to notice her weight and hair more and often criticized her image in the mirror.

A month or so passed, and she happened to see Drew again at another party. He engaged her as soon as she walked into the room; instantly attentive, Drew made sure Britney had whatever she needed that night. He asked Britney about her friends and her parents and revealed some intimate details from his own life. When a friend told Britney that her car was in a no-parking zone, Drew offered to go out and move it for her. With Drew's gaze on her, Britney felt her self-esteem soar; all of the negative feelings she had about herself, even a few hours before the party, were wiped away. She instantly felt more confident and socially outgoing and became lively and gregarious with the people around her. As a result, more people talked with her, and she felt like the life of the party. The night culminated in Britney and Drew hooking up, which seemed to Britney like the icing on the cake. The next day she felt redemption: He did in fact like her, and she no longer felt rejected by him. Each time she relived the moments of the night before, she felt buoyant and powerful. However, as time passed, so too did this temporary spike in self-esteem.

The days went by, and she did not hear from Drew, except for the occasional "whassup" in the hallway. Britney became increasingly self-critical. She withdrew from her family and excessively focused on her appearance. After another month, she saw Drew at a football game. He was interested, engaged, warm, and friendly, and Britney, just like someone who is starving for food, agreed to one more hookup. She hoped that maybe, just maybe, this time Drew would continue to be charming the next day. He was not.

As this example illustrates, the repeated hookup is damaging—it survives and endures by consuming the woman's self-esteem. Each time the woman chooses to go back for another round, she is effectively putting herself back in the line of fire. Although the repeated hookup is doomed from the start, the woman typically experiences this failure as her fault. Each time she feels rejected, another layer is taken away from her sense of self. In this way, her self-worth becomes depleted.

Often the man involved in a sextimacy encounter has no intention of being in a committed relationship with any woman, as he may not be psychologically or emotionally ready for such. Nonetheless, the woman experiences the lack of a commitment that results from such a hookup as a personal rejection of her inner self. This is primarily why she goes back for more. She is attempting to repair and make up the self-esteem deficit. Of course, the guy is still who he was a month ago, emotionally and psychologically not prepared for or capable of more than a hookup, and he behaves in the same manner he did previously. For the woman, each successive encounter contributes to an accumulating sense of personal rejection. The growing weight of this makes it more and more difficult for her to objectively see the man as he is.

THE ONE-NIGHT STAND

This sextimacy dynamic is characterized by a one-time sexual encounter with a man who is largely unknown by the woman. Although not typically what women want, the one-night stand does provide temporary self-validation. For some, the one-night stand first begins as a way for adolescents to purposely lose their virginity. This can create a template for what will become a pattern.

Many teenagers tell me they are embarrassed by their virginity and want to "get it over with." Male virginity has long been stigmatized, but there is now a growing stigma toward female virginity. Young women tell me their lack of sexual sophistication leaves them feeling left out by friends, awkward with men, and marginalized within their social network. For some, once they become labeled a virgin, they tend to be less sought out romantically. These young women are caught in a conflict between wanting to plunge forth sexually, to relieve feeling left out of the social loop, and simultaneously feeling a lack of desire or emotional preparedness for a sexual relationship. In addition, many young people have the fantasy that once they lose their virginity, they will find a boyfriend or form a committed relationship.

As fearful as they may be, these girls (and often boys, too) white-knuckle it through their first sexual encounter, all the while feeling unloved and disconnected. Their hope is that by getting their first sexual encounter over with, they will develop the confidence needed to develop a committed relationship. The result is something less desirable. The young woman leaves her first sexual encounter feeling empty, used, and completely underwhelmed by her experience. If others know of her sexual experience, then this information may easily become fodder for gossip. The young woman often feels more embarrassed and sexually awkward than she did before having sex.

The woman who engages in the one-night-stand dynamic with a series of different men often experiences social anxiety and intense feelings of self-consciousness. This sounds counterintuitive, as you might imagine that someone who is brazen enough to have sex with a person she barely knows must feel fairly self-assured. Typically, this is not the case. Individuals who are shy and inhibited expect judgment and fear they are being evaluated by others. Those with shy temperaments struggle with life changes in general. For them, starting new jobs, forging friendships, and taking on new activities often bring intense anxiety. For the shy and anxious, sex is a potentially crippling life event, as it feels like the most intimate and invasive of experiences. They cope with sexual anxiety by removing as much of the personal element as possible; this allows them to become more sexually outgoing.

The one-night stand is alluring to the socially anxious person because it involves no emotional connection, no personal banter, and no expectations, and this translates into less fear of feeling evaluated. The one-night stand is usually hasty, and the participants make a quick exit before anything becomes too emotionally messy. The anonymity of the experience helps the woman to feel sexually uninhibited.

The downside of the one-night stand is that it lays a foundation in the mind that says sex is to be disconnected from love. Over time, this can lead to tremendous difficulty enjoying sex except when it occurs separate from love and genuine care. Psychologists call this a split or disconnect between love and sex. The sex/love split occurs because our minds process, remember, and understand events according to mental schemas. Each time you engage in a new activity, the brain forms a mental schema, or road map, for that event. The first time you ride a bike, learn to swim, eat watermelon, or learn to drive, a schema forms in your mind that contains memories from those first experiences.

When you learn to drive, your mind encodes driving facts, images, and sensations. Each time you drive, your mind expects the experience to match the schema or blueprint it has of the original event. Each additional driving experience places more data within the brain's driving schema. Once driving becomes well learned and rote, you automatically, without any words or conscious thought, pull up your driving schema and drive. Sex works in a similar manner.

The way a person is first introduced to his or her sexuality—directly with romantic partners and indirectly through media, pornography, and advertising—develops a schema in his or her brain for what to expect sexually. When a woman's first sexual experiences are with partners who neither value nor know her, conditions are ready-made for sexual disconnection. A woman may find little physical pleasure and, instead, is left feeling objectified and disconnected from the person and from her own body, as if she is doing something entirely for someone else. These are the memories that are placed within the brain's sexual schema, and because they are the first, they are the most salient.

She may find that she has difficulty being sexual or experiencing pleasure with anyone with whom she is in a monogamous or committed relationship; these circumstances simply do not match her brain's mental blueprint for sex. When someone who truly cares about her shows romantic interest, it is as if the mind says, "Something is not quite right here." This thought may become consciously interpreted as, "I don't really like this guy," but what it actually means is this new data was not in the original schema for sex. The young woman, believing she is not attracted to this person who is caring toward her, moves on and chooses another one-night stand because this is a better match for her mental blueprint.

Through the years and as relationship demands grow in complexity, the woman who is prone to the one-night stand finds that a committed relationship eludes her. I have met with many women who tell me they very much want a partnership, but find it excruciatingly painful to be sexually intimate or revealing with someone who also shows a deep and genuine fondness for them. Each time a woman rejects a man who demonstrates that he genuinely wants to know her, she also loses the opportunity to broaden her romantic/sexual schema. And she learns to depend on the one-night stand in adulthood as a method of gaining male attention.

Marissa was pretty, athletic, and professionally advanced but struggled most of her life to feel accepted and liked by men. Marissa grew up in a small town, and although quite shy, she was popular and well liked. She had the same group of friends since kindergarten and so rarely had to form new relationships. As she went through her early teenage years, she felt increasingly shy and awkward around the boys in her peer group. She never felt she could be herself in front of them and much preferred to stay with her close group of female friends. Nonetheless, the guys kept appearing, and they would often make advances toward her. This male attention was painful, even mortifying to Marissa because of her shy nature.

Marissa became so anxious from the pressure of all this male attention that, in an impulsive moment and with the hope of putting the anxiety behind her, she decided to go for it and lose her virginity. Marissa's first sexual experience was on a park bench when she was fourteen years old. She recalled this experience vividly. She remembered having a tremendous amount of anxiety at the party she was attending that evening. Zack, a boy on whom she had a crush, was flirting with and engaging her. She felt overwhelmed by the attention she received and, simultaneously, believed something was wrong with her for feeling so self-conscious. All of her girlfriends seemed comfortable and excited around guys. What was wrong with her that she just wanted to be with her friends or alone? She resolved this tension by telling herself that it was normal to be with guys, that she needed to be like her friends, and that having sex would help her grow up.

Within an hour, Marissa downed three beers and was joking with her friends about sex, something she knew very little about. Each time Zack approached her, she pushed away her fear and shyness by telling herself that he must really like her. When they slipped away and did have sex, she felt empty and uncomfortable. Marissa threw up in front of Zack and was humiliated. She vowed to herself that she would tell no one. She was afraid to tell her friends because of what they may think of her. Marissa avoided Zack and cringed remembering how he had seen her in such a physically embarrassing way. She closed the book on the event and told herself to just not think about it ever again.

Through the years, high school life became more complicated for Marissa. She began to have a stronger desire for male attention and repeatedly resolved this through one-night stands. By the time Marissa was a senior in high school, she felt many of her peers "hated" her, and she frequently suffered hearing other girls whisper "slut" as she walked through her school's hallways.

Marissa excelled academically in college and went on to develop a career. By the time she came to see me, she was twenty-seven years old and deeply longed for a meaningful connection with a man. Although she had experienced success in many areas of her life, she felt the ability to form a healthy relationship was her Achilles' heel. Men asked Marissa out regularly, and they were interested in getting to know her. Nonetheless, she was unable to become intimate and comfortable with men who took her seriously and who wanted to know the real her. Marissa had become skilled at making herself whoever she imagined the men in her life wanted her to be.

Therapy involved helping Marissa to connect with her experience of herself and others, to put words to her experiences, and to fully participate in the get-to-know-you process that meaningful relationships require. Marissa had strong female friendships and, over time, learned to use with men the same type of communication she used with her female friends. It was difficult, initially, to reveal her true self to the men in her life, but with time she was pleasantly surprised to find men were interested and accepting of her deeper and more complicated self.

SEXTIMACY IS CYCLICAL

When I show the women I work with—women like Marissa, Britney, and Monica—the cyclical nature of sextimacy in a clinical and objective manner, they find they are able to gain more control over its occurrence. As they develop self-awareness for what they are experiencing in the moment, they know, well in advance, when they are about to enter sextimacy territory. This awareness enables them to detour around sextimacy and move in a more satisfying direction. Understanding this cycle helps women make fully aware sexual decisions that lead to achieving their relationship goals. There are four phases to this cycle:

1. The Depleted Self
2. The Fantasy
3. The Conquest
4. The Aftermath

The Depleted Self

There are degrees of sextimacy. But, just as bacteria thrive on a weak host, sextimacy is more likely to dominate those women who struggle the most with low self-esteem. Women who engage in chronic sextimacy tell me they feel poorly about themselves on a deep and profound level. They may face body-image issues, eating disorders, depression, and intermittent feelings of worthlessness. The reasons for these negative feelings are numerous and idiosyncratic. However, two common

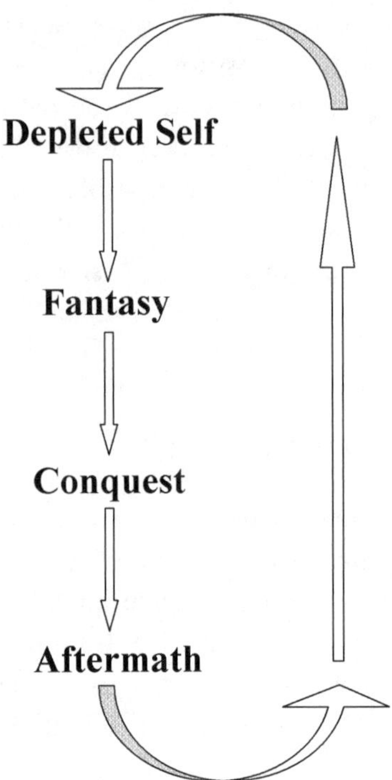

elements that will create a mild or acute depleted self are defeating parent/child interactions and faulty cultural messages about what female sexuality and female attractiveness should be.

Caregivers have a central impact on girls; they can single-handedly cause a depleted self to develop or help to relieve symptoms of a depleted self (as will be outlined in chapter 3). Parents and caregivers who do not attend to the emotional needs of their daughters set the stage for their daughters to accept one-sided relationships. From her parents a girl may learn that close relationships are not supposed to be about her needs and will then live out this lesson through her choice of romantic partners in adulthood.

Another way girls become socialized to experience a depleted self and the resulting sextimacy dynamic is through the unrealistic depiction of how sexual attractiveness is supposed to look (as explored in chapter 2). Girls and women are bombarded by visual representations that promote a sexualized image of young girls. These images and associated cultural messages communicate to women that to look sexy is to look like young girls and, equally self-defeating, that focusing on perfecting external appearance in a way that meets this standard will bring emotional fulfillment.

A particular mind-set can also foster the development of a depleted self. Women who feel their sex lives and relationships are out of control typically dislike themselves. They spend excessive time actively engaging in hard self-criticisms and hyper-focusing on their external appearance. They torture themselves over their appearance by critiquing and judging every line, roll, and perceived quirk. They may engage in repetitive thinking, constantly replaying distressing events from the past. They relive upsetting conversations, second-guessing and judging themselves for what they say or do. All of which is corrosive to their self-confidence and sense of wellbeing.

Sextimacy temporarily relieves depleted feelings about the self by offering instant self-esteem and validation. The depleted self is pivotal to the inception and continuation of sextimacy. Chapters 4 to 6 are devoted to helping women build their core selves. As many have learned, in order to form emotionally and sexually intimate relationships with men, it is essential to first develop a positive sense of self.

The Fantasy

What fills the mind with relief from the depleted self? Fantasy. Research suggests the more we actively visualize positive events occurring, the better we feel. Mindfully visualizing desired scenarios has a powerful effect on mood and even outcome. Visualization and guided imagery are techniques that therapists have long employed to help patients feel better and to gain control over dreaded future events. The more you imagine yourself handling something differently, the more likely you are to actually handle it differently when the event occurs in real time.

Unfortunately, this holds true for negative visualization, as well. Actively replaying negative scenes and memories from the past contributes to negative thinking and a depressed mood. Imagining future worst-case scenarios reduces confidence in one's ability to manage future events and contributes to feelings of hopelessness.

Invariably, when the self is depleted, the mind tends to repeat negative events and imagine negative future events. When that is the case, fantasy or daydreaming as an escape may also pave the way to sextimacy. A sextimacy fantasy typically involves the idea that male desire will deliver love, acceptance, and emotional fusion.

Women who engage in sextimacy replay romantic scenes in their minds. They may imagine someone they hook up with becoming part of a long-term relationship or imagine going on a romantic date with a sextimacy partner. For younger women, the fantasy is often that they will finally have an interaction with the object of their affection or crush. Other women fantasize about meeting Prince Charming, where sexual fireworks are lit and emotional intimacy is quick to follow.

Past sextimacy encounters are relived and become romanticized as being more meaningful than they were in reality. A woman may play out scenarios in her mind where a deeper relationship develops following the sexual act. Although this may occasionally occur for a few, for most it is an unrealistic hope. Once the sextimacy card is played, it is close to impossible to backtrack to the getting-to-know-you process of dating—a truly necessary ingredient for emotionally intimate relationships to develop. If the man is either too emotionally immature for a relationship or simply does not want a committed relationship, there is really no way to change this through sex. And, yet, the fantasy (and the relief it provides) of a meaningful relationship developing keeps the woman believing that it is a possibility, and this possibility, however slight, drives her back to another round of sextimacy.

Like a drug, fantasy pulls one out of a dark-mood state and away from a negative self-image. Fantasy allows a woman to be whomever she so desires—attractive, special, wanted. This powerful elixir contributes to the occurrence and recurrence of sextimacy events. As the woman imagines developing a bond through a sexual relationship with the object of her affection, she is also rehearsing its occurrence. Then when presented with a real-life opportunity to become sexual with the fantasy object, it is almost automatic to push forward. It is hard to say no to something once you have already prepared your mind for it; imagine eating your favorite food and then actually being presented with it. The brain is primed, the wiring is in place, and this can make saying "no" incredibly difficult.

Britney, as described earlier, was vulnerable to a repeated hookup because she felt depleted before and after her first hookup with Drew, and she actively imagined scenarios whereby she could restore her self-image through Drew's positive attention. The moment Drew approaches, even if only interested in sex, Britney sees the opportunity rehearsed in her fantasies. Her fantasies do not include Drew's failure to exhibit any interest in getting to know her on a deeper level. She is unable to assess Drew's capacity for relationship development and is unable to see that what he is offering is sex alone.

In chapter 7, we will look at the importance of exploring a person's history with love as a starting place to building a new, more fulfilling love pattern. As the women I work with gain sharp awareness for whom they choose to have sex with and how they may repeat certain problematic dynamics from their background, they create a road map showing them where to travel romantically and what spots to avoid.

The Conquest

For some women the conquest, or sexual act itself, is intense, as it merges the core desires of the depleted self with elements of fantasy. The depleted self is replaced by a powerful self that briefly feels special and cherished. The powerful self is momentarily filled with feelings of euphoria, acceptance, desirability, and worthiness. The rush of adrenaline, the release of oxytocin and other neurotransmitters is so overwhelming that a mistaken meaning is derived that this ephemeral chemistry is a real and enduring connection.

On the other hand, for many women and for young women in particular, when sextimacy is involved, the conquest is neither sexually stimulating nor sexually pleasing. Because enjoyable sex for women is typically a byproduct of both mind and body, sextimacy leaves them feeling disappointed and unfulfilled. They are often not full participants in their sexual experiences and tend to check out during their encounters. While the sexual encounter is occurring, the woman feels disconnected and alone in her experience. This represents the worst-case scenario because not only does the woman have to manage a self-defeating sextimacy event, but she is also disconnecting from her body. This coping strategy is entirely contrary to developing a healthy self-image or a pleasurable sexual life.

When sextimacy begins in the teenage years, it leaves a young woman with little freedom to fully develop and understand her sexuality. If a pattern of unfulfilling, disconnected sexual encounters continues, it becomes difficult to forge emotionally intimate, sexually fulfilling relationships with men in adulthood. In chapter 8, we will turn to the work of helping women understand their sexual selves. When women explore and develop an understanding of their sexuality separate from pleasing men, they more easily connect with sexual pleasure and generally have a more fulfilling sex life.

Whether the sexual conquest in sextimacy is intense or detached, it is typically quick. Yet, the event itself has an enduring and profound impact on how the woman sees herself and her ability to get what she ultimately wants from men.

The Aftermath

When sextimacy is involved, what should be an afterglow of warmth and positive wellbeing rapidly turns to disappointment. The glow disappears, and feelings of the depleted self return, only these negative feelings are often stronger and harsher than they were previously. When sex occurs with an unfamiliar partner, the aftermath is typically characterized by a feeling of awkwardness.

For men, this may cause them to want to flee and to flee soon. For women, it can lead to intense feelings of self-consciousness and wondering if they are being critically evaluated by their partner. A kind of anxious energy permeates, whereby the woman may begin to ask questions to relieve this tension: "What should we do now? . . . What is your type? . . . What kind of girls do you like? . . . Dinner tonight? . . . A cup of coffee?" For the man, this anxious energy only heightens his sense of feeling trapped and his need for a quick escape. If at his locale, he makes the woman feel so awkward that she leaves. If at a neutral locale, he chats some and then makes his exit. Some women beat the man to the punch, quickly decamping before they catch the slightest hint of rejection.

Either way, soon after the sextimacy partner is gone, for many women, self-consciousness gives way to self-loathing, and the depleted self comes roaring back. Now the woman is left not only with her original set of harsh self-criticisms, but also an additional set that has to do with feeling taken advantage of and sexually used. Although women are initially willing participants in sextimacy, in the end they often feel used because they are fantasizing and hoping for more than sex alone. The realization that it was just a sexual event for the man leaves the woman feeling hurt and not good enough to get what she truly desires. Of course, it is not the woman who is worthless. The problem is a flawed strategy. Sextimacy, by and large, does not foster committed, monogamous love.

So the woman is left with unbearable feelings of worthlessness, making her vulnerable to fantasy as a means of escape, which, of course, leads to more instances of sextimacy. Some women, on the other hand, cope with the aftermath by telling themselves that it was *they* who used the man. These women drink the Kool-Aid, so to speak (as outlined in chapter 8), and work hard to convince themselves that all they really want is a sexual hookup.

CONCLUSION

Women repeatedly tell me they are seeking meaningful, committed, emotionally intimate, and sexually fulfilling relationships with men. They crave emotional closeness and an enduring, reliable sense of contentment. Sextimacy is in opposition to these goals and is a cycle of continually dating men who confirm a woman's negative self-image. In order to gain control over this dynamic, it is important to both identify when sextimacy is occurring and what the underlying factors are that contribute to its occurrence.

In the next two chapters, we will explore cultural and family factors that condition many women to settle for sextimacy and forgo their true goal of emotional intimacy. Then we turn to the work of helping women build stronger relationships with themselves through increased emotional awareness, direct communication, and self-esteem development. In the final three chapters, we will explore how women who struggle with sextimacy may use this self-knowledge to achieve their sexual and relationship goals.

SELF-ASSESSMENT: ARE YOU A SEXTIMACY JUNKIE?

After reading this chapter, you may wonder if you have a sextimacy issue or if you are in the clear. Here is a self-assessment to help you determine your sextimacy ratio. The more items you endorse, the more you turn to sextimacy for a quick fix.

1. Do you feel empty after sex or hooking up?
2. Do you have sex or hook up soon after meeting someone new?
3. Do you find that most of the time you spend with your romantic partners occurs before or while hooking up?
4. Do you feel energized when a man shows sexual interest in you and then let down after the sexual event?
5. Do you feel inhibited and guarded around men when forced to deal with them in nonsexual contexts?
6. Do you find that your relationships often begin passionately but cool quickly?
7. Do you think your partners enjoy sex or hooking up more than you do?
8. Do you use sex as a way to get emotionally closer to men and then feel let down and disappointed when it does not occur?
9. Have you had more sexual or hookup partners than you are comfortable admitting?
10. Do you find that you do not know your partners well before having sex or hooking up?
11. Do you feel less attracted to men who ask you out or who directly express interest in getting to know you?
12. Do you find that you are sexual with men you do not know well but emotionally close to those you do not find physically attractive?
13. Was your first sexual experience with someone you did not know well and did not later get to know well?

14. Did the caregivers (men in particular) in your life take little interest in getting to know you emotionally?
15. Have you agreed to sex or hooking up to quell feelings of loneliness as opposed to true sexual desire?
16. Do you have sex or hook up hoping that it will open the door to getting to know the person better and a future relationship?
17. Do you have trouble being alone or *not* having a "crush" on someone?
18. Do you feel awkward and self-conscious after having sex or hooking up?
19. Have you never experienced a sexual relationship with a man who has also truly known you?
20. Do you use flirting to the exclusion of other avenues for getting to know the men you are romantically interested in, such as participating in activities together, dating, friendship, shared interests, and intellectual discussions?

2

Perfect Little Dolls

Cultural and Societal Factors

Women, at least in the developed world, are less dependent on men than ever before in history. And yet, women remain dependent on and controlled by men in many ways. Although they have more choices and freedoms, they are more depressed. Do women have it all for the first time in history, or have they put themselves in a box, hemmed in by even more things at which they need to be perfect? It is no longer acceptable to only look young when you *are* young; now seventy is the new fifty. It is no longer enough to appear chaste and virginal; now young women must simultaneously appear seductive and innocent. It is not enough to only work or to only raise children; many women now have several children while simultaneously serving as the primary breadwinner. The perfectionistic messages geared toward women are astounding, and it is easy to wonder how women do all of this and how they do it all so effectively. In an effort to meet such expectations and maintain an image of perfection, many successful women cope by subtly disconnecting from themselves. Those who take this path become little dolls, doing all that is expected of them without actually experiencing their lives.

In this chapter, we explore how the current cultural context influences girls' development with contradictory messages and contributes to them becoming women who disconnect from the reality of their lives. This disconnect can make it difficult for a woman to develop an authentic sense of herself and can leave her vulnerable to sextimacy. The same milieu leads girls to develop an external focus at the expense of their interior lives. Girls and women who see themselves only through the eyes of others have limited knowledge of their own needs. Without the capacity to recognize their own true feelings, women cannot successfully pursue personal happiness.

Even with the best of intentions by parents and caregivers, girls are still developing their sexual identities in a world that encourages disconnecting from the self. This disavowal begins in girlhood and may persist for a lifetime, making women vulnerable to losing touch with their sexual selves and to using sextimacy as a substitute for real intimacy. The culture abounds with messages that take women further away from their goal of authentic relationships with others and toward a fragmented sense of self. The tricky part is that these messages appear to offer appealing, easy ways to develop a sense of closeness with others, and many women come to believe they represent a shortcut to intimacy and contentment.

BIOLOGY PRECEDES EMOTIONAL DEVELOPMENT

Girls are intimately in tune with parental and societal expectations. As they negotiate these complicated social demands, they also must manage physical and biological changes before they are cognitively and emotionally ready. Joan Jacobs Brumberg, social historian and author of *The Body Project*, notes that in the 1800s, menarche, or first menstruation, typically occurred around the ages of fifteen to sixteen. Currently, menarche is more likely to occur around the age of twelve. Brumberg attributes this younger menarche to economic progress—better living conditions, less malnutrition, and less disease. In order to menstruate, girls must have a certain body fat ratio; therefore, better diets and less disease have contributed to girls weighing more than they did even thirty years ago. In many ways, earlier menarche is a sign of better health. There is a discrepancy, however, as Brumberg argues, in that biological development does not coincide with emotional or cognitive development. Although girls begin to have the biological functions of adult women and appear more womanly, they are still girls in terms of their cognitive and emotional maturity.[1] At the age of twelve, girls have difficulty separating their thoughts and feelings from those of others and may experience the feelings of others as if they are their own. Young girls are still developing problem-solving and judgment skills, and typically they struggle in terms of thinking through the long-term consequences for a particular decision or predicament. These areas of cognitive development are pivotal to understanding sexuality and for managing sexual behaviors in a healthy manner.

However, modern Western culture does not allow girls much time for their cognitive development to catch up with their physical development. Parents, media, schools, and teachers treat girls who outwardly appear womanly as if they are women. Girls have little, if any, space to catch up and to explore their sexuality in a safe and boundaried manner. On the day a girl starts her first period, she has the same sense of herself as she did the day before, and yet, she aptly and intuitively notices how different her life has become. She sees her own image in advertisements portraying young girls looking sexually provocative, she senses her parents treating her more protectively and questioning her intentions, and she sees men looking at her in ways that confuse and intrigue her. This thrust into adulthood is an abrupt loss of innocence, which often takes with it the young girl's burgeoning sense of self.

There was a time when girls had the luxury of more time before the onset of puberty and also experienced increased female support. According to Brumberg, in the late nineteenth century, many all-girl groups were formed in order to nurture the female through the adolescent period. Girls routinely spent time each week in Girl Scouts, Campfire Girls, 4-H, and female religious or church groups. In these groups, they were mentored by women of various ages. This allowed girls to connect with others, feel a sense of belonging, provide and receive care, and gain a sense of acceptance. These needs are inherently tied to female identity and are piercingly present during adolescent development.[2] As Brumberg points out, although many same-sex groups also were repressive, these groups did offer a safe and healthy buffer for the development of an identity. Young girls continue to have these basic core needs, but far fewer healthy outlets exist today, and by puberty many girls opt out of the organized same-sex groups that are available. Instead, as adolescents, girls look to the consumer culture to provide a sense of acceptance and belonging.

In the span of a few months, many adolescent girls are lost to the glossy images they see in magazines and movies and begin to substitute a sense of self with working to appear like these images.[3] At this stage, these messages impact girls almost immediately, and naturally, they begin to believe that they are, in fact, women. As a result, adolescent girls are more likely to make unsafe decisions about sex that may lead to sextimacy events, pregnancy, and the risk of sexually transmitted diseases (STDs).

At the same time, internally, most adolescent girls still feel like little girls and are often overwrought with confusion and angst about how to understand themselves sexually and emotionally. This conflict is seen by parents who are confused when their pubescent daughters at one moment want their "mommy's attention" and at another dress in a sexy manner to go to the mall. Parents are alarmed when their girls make a seemingly sudden transition from girlhood to womanhood. As a result of fear and confusion and in an effort to protect, parents may unknowingly contribute to the objectification of their daughters.

THE CULTURE OF PARENTS

Cultural messages, delivered by public media, peers, teachers, and other parents, not only seduce pubescent girls but also their parents. The message is clear to parents: Your baby is all grown up, and you better get used to it. Fathers and mothers typically have different ways of responding to their adolescent daughters, ways that are often reflective of their own misguided sexual experiences in adolescence and young adulthood. Fathers take on the role of conditioning their daughters to become sexual gatekeepers. Many mothers, on the other hand, encourage their daughters to attract male attention, while giving mixed messages about commitment and little guidance to understanding their emotional worlds. This creates a mindbender where an adolescent girl focuses on becoming a sexually appealing gatekeeper who has no sounding board for her new, more complicated emotional self.

Many fathers feel anxious about their daughters' transition to adolescents, and their communications begin to take on a moralistic tone: "Should," "Should Not," "Right," "Wrong," "Good," "Bad." Fathers begin to say things like, "Your top is too short . . . Why are you wearing that? . . . Only a certain kind of girl wears that kind of shirt . . . Your pants are too tight," and the list goes on. The anxious communications of many fathers to their developing daughters suggest that girls should be a "certain way" and are inviting "problems," presumably pregnancy, rape, or STDs, if they do not handle themselves in this "good way."[4] These messages implicitly convey to girls that they should be hypervigilant to the signals they are putting out to men through their appearance, attitude, flirtations, and general behavior. These messages also suggest that the daughter is the sexual gatekeeper, and if something bad should happen to her, it is her fault. Amidst these confusing messages, the young girl is searching to form an identity and now feels yet another loss, as her father no longer treats her as he did before she was an adolescent. In addition, she sees no viable alternatives for her happiness; she can either please her father or please potential male partners.

Many fathers inadvertently project their own experiences as adolescent boys and men onto their young daughters. By doing this, they miss a wealth of important information about what is actually important to their daughters. They only scratch the surface in communicating about appearance and do not plunge deeper or attempt to understand their daughters' innermost feelings and anxieties. Many fathers give their girls the idea that what is most important about them is that they appear sufficiently chaste and comport themselves as a "good girl" should. This can be stifling for the developing girl who may react either by rebelling through sextimacy or by developing a repressed and pent-up sexual self. This male model often repeats in that the girl is likely to pick a partner who is repressive and judgmental of her sexuality.

Culture creates dilemmas for mothers about how best to protect their developing daughters. Some feel caught in a bind between wanting their daughters to be desired by men while simultaneously fearing they will become "fast," "loose," and get a "reputation." They often resolve this anxiety by focusing their young girls' attention on attaining a boyfriend and maintaining relationships. This conditioning begins early in female development by mothers who quiz their daughters about love interests in a way that communicates to girls that having a boyfriend is, above all else, the most important thing they can do. They may ask their daughters, even at ages eight or nine, "Who is your boyfriend?" or "Whom do you like in your class?" and they may begin to ask if their daughter saw the particular person that day. As their daughters get older, it can feel like a status symbol for many mothers if the girl dates someone well thought of in their community. Mothers will ask their daughters about their friends' romantic relationships, almost as a way to see where their daughters stand in the social hierarchy: "Does Sue have a boyfriend *yet*?" Mothers also pummel their daughters with questions about particular love interests: "When are you and Josh going out again? . . . When are you going to meet Josh's parents?" or "Where is Josh going to college? . . . Maybe we can have Josh over for dinner on Sunday." There is anxiety and pressure involved in this line of questioning, which communicates to the girl that there is something scary about not having a boyfriend, and therefore, finding and maintaining a man should be the major focus of her attention.

Mothers fail to acknowledge to their daughters (although not usually to themselves) that, in order to maintain romantic relationships at such a young age, their daughters are typically sexually active without any true enjoyment of the sex act itself. When, finally, a daughter asks for birth control, these mothers will feign surprise and lecture about the possibility, if not too careful, of being classified as a "slut." When daughters talk about a conflict or breach in connection with a guy, these mothers will point out how the daughter should fix the problem or what she may have done wrong. In these cases, mothers are unknowingly reinforcing the message to their daughters that their value is in their ability to maintain relationships with men.

At the other end of the spectrum are mothers who do not provide their daughters with the protection of healthy boundaries and unwittingly promote their daughters' promiscuity. What in the past was dressing one's daughter up for a gentleman caller is now allowing the daughter to spend the night at a coed sleepover. "How could

I say no, all of her friends will be there?" Unlike those mothers who overemphasize the importance of relationships, these mothers tend to promote autonomy at any cost. They encourage their daughters to be self-sufficient, high achieving, and focused on school. When it comes to relationships, they offer superficial "independent woman" rhetoric, including "Play the field," "You don't have time for relationships," and "Never depend on a man." This cynicism dismisses the importance of relationships to girls, and later to women, who then begin to see sextimacy as a way to connect without the pressure of a real relationship. The oversimplification of the intense need girls have for relationships and the lack of helpful advice about managing their emotional worlds leave girls with no road map for how to merge passion with intimacy.

Given our culture's mistreatment of women who do not appear traditionally feminine or attractive, many mothers also have tremendous anxiety concerning their daughters' physical appearance. These mothers want their daughters to feel accepted and self-confident and believe improving their appearance will help. Well before their daughters even tune into physical appearance, many mothers offer their girls makeup or suggest a way to lose weight. The implicit message is that these girls are not enough on their own and that perfecting their physical appearance is essential to finding love. Daughters come to believe they will be evaluated in the same way by the men in their lives and thus remain ever vigilant should physical shortcomings be exposed.

The confusing messages parents give their daughters blur the landscape, leaving girls with little direction in terms of how to understand their emotional worlds or how to develop mutually loving relationships. Quite to the contrary, a protective factor for girls in developing their sexuality, and forming long-term relationships, is having access to at least one adult who offers an understanding, nonjudgmental point of view about female sexuality. Rather than surface messages about physical appearance or "getting a reputation," what helps girls most is when parents talk to their daughters in such a way that invites daughters to consider their *own* feelings and perspectives regarding sex.[5]

Coming of age in our current culture leaves many girls with few healthy outlets to express or understand their sexuality and increasing desire for male connection. Instead, an adolescent girl is often left to feel she cannot trust her mother because when she attempts to express her deeper, more complicated self, her perspective is dismissed or criticized. In her relationship with her father, she learns that girls are responsible when bad things happen and so are not to be trusted. Over time, many girls adapt by embracing a stance that says if you can't beat them, join them, which means they turn on one another.

GIRLS AGAINST GIRLS

Historically, the world in general communicates to women from birth that they are not quite enough on their own and that they must work hard to make up the difference. It was not so long ago that it was acceptable for family and friends to express disappointment over the birth of a girl. Some women were made to feel inadequate if they birthed a girl, and many would publicly hope their next would be a boy. Albeit on a far more restrained level, this bias still exists. When I was pregnant with my son, more than one person remarked, "It is good to have a boy first." This inexplicable counsel is a disappointing reminder that girls are still not fully valued.

Women continue to be brutalized in order to be good enough for men. In parts of Africa, little girls endure female circumcision in an effort to ensure their premarital virginity. In the United States, some women go to great lengths (some may even say self-mutilate) through plastic surgery to become more pleasing to men and in the process suffer considerable emotional distress and physical pain. As a consequence of being treated as if something essential is missing from their very nature, many women operate with the belief that other women must also be deficient.

Early in puberty, girls begin to look at one another in an acutely competitive and judgmental manner. Many come to see each other as competitors for the attraction of boys and men. They tend to blame one another when bad things happen to them, just as they have been taught to blame themselves. If mistreated by a guy, other girls will comment, "Well, she is a slut" or "I told her he was cheating on her." When attracted to a guy who already has a girlfriend, girls often find ways to attack their competitor's character or appearance. They may comment on the sexual exploits of other girls, casually referring to them as "skanks" or "whores" to describe their nature. If a boyfriend or a hookup cheats, many girls (and adult women, too) find it easier to blame the other woman than actually hold the male accountable.

Our culture stigmatizes women who do not meet traditional standards of beauty, and too often, women use this unforgiving reality to harshly judge one another as a means to gain leverage and power. Many girls struggle with body hatred and tend to project their own self-hatred onto other girls. For example, girls tend to compare body sizes or when they feel let down by a girlfriend, will console themselves with "Well, at least I am not as fat as she is."

In a world that feels as if others could turn on you at any time, taking a judgmental stance toward other women is a way for women to feel a modicum of control. Judging the physical appearance of others allows some women to hold on to the belief that if they do things right and look good, they will be safe and their relationships will endure. The cost of this tactic is high because harsh judgment and cruelty toward other women is inherently tied to relentless self-scrutiny and panic should their own flaws be attacked.

In her eye-opening book *Odd Girl Out*, Rachel Simmons, an expert in the area of female aggression, interviewed adolescent girls from several regions of the country about their experiences with relational aggression or female bullying. Simmons began her meetings with various groups of girls by asking the same question: "What are some of the differences between the ways guys and girls are mean?" Girls responded with descriptors such as "Girls are secretive . . . They destroy you from the inside . . . Girls are manipulative . . . There's an aspect of evil in girls that isn't in boys . . . Girls target you where they know you're weakest . . . Girls do a lot behind each other's backs . . . Girls plan and premeditate . . . With guys, you know where you stand . . . I feel a lot safer with guys."[6] Reading these descriptors, you might think these girls were talking about a group of antisocial criminals. Many girls see one another as scary, untrustworthy, ruthless, and cruel.

In Simmons's research, she finds that girls are paralyzed and panicked by female bullying, including such behaviors as ganging up on one another, giving the evil eye, gossiping, shunning, ignoring, and a host of other disparaging acts. When Simmons asked, "What is it like when another girl glares at you?", an adolescent girl responded, "It makes you feel lower and deteriorates your insides. Oh God, you think, what are they doing? You ask them why they're mad, and they don't say anything. You have no control. It gives them power."[7] Girls who are the victims of female bullying feel painfully confused, as they are given no direct information as to what caused the rift in the relationship.

Girls often form their own sort of closure by developing an internal, self-critical monologue about what they did to cause the falling out. As one ostracized teenage girl told me while trying to make sense of why all of her girlfriends suddenly stopped talking to her, "I am not sure what it is yet, but I must have a fatal character flaw that will keep ruining my relationships." This type of self-critical response depletes adolescent girls' self-esteem to the point of depression. The 2010 Massachusetts case involving the suicide of fifteen-year-old Phoebe Prince was linked to a three-month campaign of emotional and physical bullying by nine of her peers, seven of whom were girls.[8] It is believed that this unrelenting torture was inflicted on Phoebe because of upset over her dating relationship with a popular male peer.

Why do girls do this to one another? Girls, and many women, believe they must conform to a rigid mold so as to maintain membership in their social groups. The mold is restrictive and ultrafeminine, as Simmons outlines: "They are the rules of femininity: girls must be modest, self-abnegating, and demure; girls must be nice and put others before themselves; girls get power by who likes them, who approves, who they know, but not by their own hand."[9]

According to Simmons, a girl who does not adhere to these rules easily becomes labeled as a girl who believes she is "all that," which translates to being assertive, self-confident, sexually secure, and less prone to self-sacrifice. An all-that girl sounds eerily similar to a girl who knows herself; however, this can be cause for punishment in the current social milieu. All-that girls often become the targets of female bullying and acts of relational aggression by other girls. Female bullying uses relationships as a weapon, and the girls who are the victims are left without the connections and nurturance that are central to their identity and sense of wellbeing.

Research suggests there is one clearly protective element in female development and that is the power of strong female relationships.[10] By judging, fearing, and excluding their own sex, women effectively self-sabotage their opportunity for strong female relationships. A self-fulfilling prophecy manifests whereby women begin to see that other women are untrustworthy. Women tend to catalog this emergence as more evidence to the nature of women and fail to consider the impact their own actions have on other women.

Girls who are fearful of one another and have fewer intimate female relationships are more likely to turn to sextimacy as an avenue for acceptance. Without the protective element of close female friendship, they feel abandoned and look for what they can control. In a world that does not value the direct expression of the complicated, messier emotions they experience, many young women have found a way to gain grounding and purpose. The energy needed for developing a sense of self becomes directed toward securing male desire through perfecting the external.

NARCISSISTIC CULTURE

The culture found a market in the self-conscious adolescent who does not know herself, her body, or how to manage her newfound physicality. A place to dock all of this insecurity is in sight—perfect your external appearance. Success in this pursuit offers temporary relief from negative emotion because it means you can do something. Taking action when distressed is universally soothing. Girls learn to direct their ambivalence and despair toward, as Brumberg terms it, "The Body Project." This ongoing ordeal requires great vigilance and painful self-consciousness but provides a clear purpose—one not as vague as "developing a sense of self." Focusing on the external to quell the internal continues into womanhood, where many tend to focus on changing something about their appearance or social status, instead of confronting what distresses them on a deeper, emotional level.

Many women engage in one colossal, never-ending self-makeover project. This lifelong makeover allows some to feel relief when they face a loss of self-esteem over a discrepancy between who they are and who they believe they should be. This applies without much regard to how a loss of self-esteem should occur. It could be the result of a divorce, a disappointing affair, a cheating boyfriend, a child in jeopardy, or a job loss. But the makeover, in effect, may amplify a woman's belief that she is entirely to blame for all that goes wrong in her life.

Self-help books and magazines are replete with tactics that tell women what they did wrong to cause their partner to cheat, that offer rules for finding and attracting a good marital partner, and that show ways to trim their waistlines and to be better lovers to the men in their lives. There are many direct physical solutions including Botox, liposuction, breast augmentation, nose jobs, porcelain veneers, vaginal rejuvenation, Restylane injections, hair extensions, fake eyelashes, and foot surgery. The list is long; name your flaw, and it can be corrected. Alcohol and drugs are romanticized, offering women easy means to dampen societal expectations and relief from the straitjacket of having to please others. And, of course, too often women mistakenly use dieting as a tool for achieving self-acceptance. Many women affix their mood to how close to perfect their reflection appears to them. If their weight is less than expected, it may feel like a blissful day and if more than expected, a horribly torturous day.

We are bombarded by images demonstrating that exposing a little extra skin will deliver romance and keeping one's skin taut will deliver years of happiness with men. All of this is done to sooth internal woes. The messages may border on the exhibitionistic, including waxing the entire vulva into a prepubescent souvenir, placing a G-string above the pant line so that it can be inspected by the public, and installing a stripper pole at home for "parties." The greater the self-esteem deficit, the more extreme the measures these women are willing to embrace to make up the difference.

This kind of narcissistic attention to the external as opposed to the internal has not always been the case. Weight became a mainstream concern for women in the 1920s when home scales became more commonplace. Before this advancement, it was more difficult to check body weight, as scales were only present at drug stores or county fairs.[11] Mirrors were not readily accessible and only became part of the middle-class home at the end of the nineteenth century. As Brumberg notes, "By the turn of the century, running water, mirrors, and electric lights provided middle-class girls with vast opportunities for self scrutiny, especially of their skin and hair."[12] These advancements allowed our culture to emphasize the importance of perfectly manicured nails and deemphasize the importance of developing a strong core self. Now it is not uncommon for girls as young as eight or nine to notice their weight and to even begin dieting.

These cultural messages implicitly tell women that a depleted mood may be traded for happiness, as long as they are willing to rework, remake, and redo their appearance. Working to perfect the self becomes an identity that supplies endless purpose. Ultimately the ongoing, excessive makeover project is self-destructive, but in the moment, these strategies and tactics can feel like a life vest. Over the long run, heeding narcissistic impulses means countless scarrings of self. As they morph themselves into display dolls, many girls and women lose touch with what actually drives their happiness.

OBJECT OF DESIRE

Advertising is the background noise of our lives, and similar to the sound of a creaking door you no longer hear, we are habituated to the barrage of billboards, magazine ads, Internet signage, and reality television that permeates. Consumers report that they do not believe advertising impacts their choices, how they see themselves, or their goals.[13] However, ads are designed to ensure that consumers do not recognize their full impact. Advertising and media agencies employ psychologists and social experts to tailor images and products to meet the innermost needs and vulnerabilities of the individual consumer. This kind of tailoring reached a new dimension with recent technology called digital signage. This system scans your face and from this image, gleans idiosyncratic data about you, including your age and gender. The technology instantaneously matches your data with general interests for your demographic. Perhaps in the near future, you may notice as you walk through the subway or an airport that ads are popping up specifically tailored to your areas of interest.

Media often convince consumers to buy a product or to look a certain way because it is associated with a fix for some perceived flaw.

Although there is a range of flaws that media tap into, girls and young women are particularly drawn to messages about finding and keeping a suitor. By offering products and images that are paired with a relationship of some sort, vulnerable girls and women begin to associate looking a certain way with finding love. As a result, many girls and women want to appear similar to the women they see in advertising.

There is a conflicting female image offered in the media, one that is neither attainable nor truly representative of the real human experience. As Jean Kilbourne, the wonderful writer and researcher in the area of women's portrayal in advertising, observes:

> Females have long been divided into virgins and whores, of course. What is new is that girls are now supposed to embody both within themselves. This is symbolic of the central contradiction of the culture—we must work hard to produce and achieve success and yet, at the same time, we are encouraged to live impulsively, spend a lot of money, and be constantly immediately gratified. This tension is reflected in our attitudes toward many things, including sex and eating. Girls are promised fulfillment both through being thin and through eating rich foods, just as they are promised fulfillment through being innocent and virginal and through wild and impulsive sex.[14]

Girls and women develop unconscious beliefs that they can be two contradictory images at one time, and then they expend their energy trying to do so. In her book *The Lolita Effect*, Gigi Durham, PhD, professor of journalism and mass communication, explores how images within the media purport certain "beauty myths" that undermine a girl's ability to develop a healthy sexual identity. These beauty myths include the following: It is important to appear sexy even at a very young age; if you work hard enough, you can look like a sex goddess; it is desirable to look simultaneously like a young girl and also like a sex kitten; violence against women is sexy; and girls should learn what boys like, so they will be more sexually desirable to them.[15] A quick perusal through popular women's or celebrity-gossip magazines confirms the prevalence of these myths.

Without question, relationships between men and women are not portrayed in the media as mutually sexually beneficial and all too often focus more on pleasing men than on pleasing women. Women's magazines provide numerous articles that primarily instruct women on the art of male seduction. Some popular articles in high-selling magazines include:[16]

> "Our Most Sizzling Sex Survey: 12,000 Men Confess What Makes Their Toes Curl. Even We Were Shocked."
> "The 7 Best Sex Tips You've Ever Heard: Bed-Tested, Couple-Approved Ideas—Try Them!"
> "Your Guy's Body: 4 Secret Pleasure Trails Every Man Has (Take a Private Tour Tonight!)"
> "Guys Tell What's Sexy (and Not Sexy) in Bed"
> "What's Your Limit for Infidelity?"
> "141 Sexy Confessions from Men about You: In Bed, at Work, Dressed, Undressed"
> "His Butt: What the Size, Shape, and Pinchability of Those Sweet Cheeks Reveal about His True Self"

A study of college-aged women showed that many are drawn to these magazines and articles because they focus on sex and the single life.[17] These publications often provide a step-by-step guide for how to become more pleasing to men, leaving the female reader with a pressing need to act on the superficial suggestions and advice. But the glow from shopping trips, makeovers, hot hookups, and other quick-fix tactics does not last. And as it fades, so too does the relief in securing a dating instruction manual.

Girls and women find these materials compelling because they are socialized to have empathy and to easily take on the perspectives of others, including those of men. The connection they are working so hard to develop, however, is to a product or a sex act and not an authentic relationship with another human being.[18] Over the long term, these artificial connections leave the woman with a lack of self-acceptance and no outlet for developing an enduring sense of internal fulfillment.

Young women are exposed to artificial connections in popular television and reality shows that present love and sex in an objectified and cynical manner. Mike Fleiss, executive producer/creator of *The Bachelor*,

ABC's popular reality show where multiple women vie for the affection of one hotly desired man, told media outlets that the typical *Bachelor* contestant has sex with three women on the show. When asked who held the record for the most sex on the show, Fleiss responded, "That's my man, Bob Guiney . . . I think it was five and a half."[19]

Where are the needs and desires of women in these programs? Men are often portrayed as having to do little more than smile or provide beer and women follow (an equally unrealistic depiction that sets men up for disappointment). Women, on the other hand, must be constant students: studying up on sexology, working to perfect their appearance, morphing themselves into sexy schoolgirls, and developing ways to be titillating bedroom conversationalists. There is little about how to form an emotionally intimate and sexually fulfilling relationship. This leaves girls and women with massive gaps in their understanding of sex and partnership from *their* perspective.

The male perspective has become so institutionalized that many women automatically view themselves from this perspective and even look at other women from the male perspective.[20] A woman experiences herself by channeling the scrutiny with which she imagines a male figure might evaluate her; she appraises herself as an object, just as she would a piece of art in a gallery. As a result of this conditioning, many women have little sense of what drives *them* sexually and engage sex with a disconnected and checked-out state of mind. A hyper-focus on the external makes it hard for a woman to understand or enjoy herself sexually from inside her own head. As Kilbourne reflects, "How sexy can a woman be who hates her body? She can act sexy, but can she feel sexy? How fully can she surrender to passion if she is worried that her thighs are too heavy or her stomach too round, if she can't bear to be seen in the light, or if she doesn't like the fragrance of her own genitals?"[21]

Most young women have very little space in which they may experience their sexuality in a safe manner that allows them to experiment, understand, and explore who they are as sexual beings. Instead, they are bombarded by contradictory messages about sexuality that suggest they are to appear perfectly, seductively innocent. Popular culture does not provide models of mutual relationships, where women are benefiting in ways other than being objects of desire.

SEXTIMACY LINK

One of the ways women navigate the cultural conundrum of being an innocent and seductive object of desire is through sextimacy. Sextimacy offers women an outlet to connect with men while still neglecting their own sexuality. After all, within a sextimacy encounter, a young woman can appear both chaste and sexy, for example, saying things like, "I do not even know you . . . I don't usually do this," while becoming intimate. In addition, sextimacy occurs as isolated events, offering a baseline of not being sexually active with peaks that can be denied and blinked away. The young woman may wake up the next day surprised by the sextimacy event and even pledge to herself not to do it again: "I will never do that type of thing again" or "I was drunk." In this way, sextimacy splits sexuality from the rest of a woman's experience of herself.

Deborah Tolman, professor of human sexuality, interviewed adolescent girls about their experience of sexual desire. One of the young women interviewed, Trisha, aptly describes this phenomenon: "I'll just have a few drinks, I mean, to the point where I get flirty, 'cause I won't do it if I'm straight. I have to wait till I get flirty, and then I'll just say, let's go . . . and then I can blame it on the alcohol and say, oh, it was because I was drunk."[22] Sextimacy allows a woman to comport herself as a "good girl" by day, and then, under certain conditions or with certain people, she may allow herself to be a "bad girl."

Girls and women fear the social death that can ensue from being labeled a "slut" by their peers. Sextimacy offers relief from this fear, as the woman can report as little or as much as she wishes to friends, and she does not have to report the sextimacy event to imagined, future romantic partners. It is equivalent to losing your wallet; it is a fluke, and there is no need to tell everyone in your life that you lost your wallet, as it will likely not happen again. On the other hand, if the event turns into a real relationship, she has achieved her fantasy. In addition, because in a sextimacy event the two people do not see each other outside of the sexual lead-up and event itself, it is quite easy for the woman to tell herself that it was a random act of passion that will not repeat. It is contradictory, but this behavior allows the woman to feel in control of her sexuality.

Many young women report that sextimacy is, quite simply, the modern single scene, as this is the main venue for women and men to connect socially. Kathleen Bogle, a sociologist, interviewed college students regarding hooking up and dating practices on college campuses.[23] The students she interviewed reported that usually after a hookup, a relationship does not develop, and in all probability, the two never see one another again. Most importantly, Bogle's research suggests that the man typically holds the power in the hookup relationship, and it is he who decides if the relationship will go any further. Bogle found that men generally do not want a hookup to turn into a meaningful relationship. Women report that they typically hope a hookup will turn into a meaningful relationship and, in some cases, initiate conversations with the man involved about deepening the connection. Sextimacy unilaterally meets the needs of men more so than women, and women are willing participants because they believe it is their only way to connect with men.

Tolman found a similar connection and observes, "We have effectively desexualized girls' sexuality, substituting the desire for relationship and emotional connection for sexual feelings in their bodies."[24] Sextimacy tends to dull the emotional intimacy right out of a sexual experience so that it becomes like a superficial reenactment of images seen in ads, pornography, or popular culture. This reenactment leaves little room for in-the-moment mutual intimacy and acting on one's inner desire. Girls and women feel invisible, not physically, but emotionally—almost as if they are not really there. Nonetheless, there are multiple social dilemmas for young women that force them to settle for disconnected and unfulfilling sexual experiences.

Some women believe they are not really supposed to enjoy sex or to see it from their own perspective, as it is somehow subversive or dirty to do so. For example, Tolman found that although most of the girls in her study experienced sexual desire, they had to sacrifice aspects of themselves to keep this desire within the acceptable limits of femininity. Some girls reported a fear of feeling desire and still being considered feminine enough to have relationships, while others reported a fear that if something unsafe occurs in the context of sexual desire, they will be at fault for actually wanting the sex. Other girls reported a fear of being branded a "slut" if they enjoy sex or, alternatively, a "prude" if they are not sexual enough. In addition, the young women Tolman interviewed had difficulty finding their voices and communicating about their sexuality in a meaningful way. Many of these girls had never previously explored, on a nuanced level, what their own sexuality meant to them. This lack of sexual exploration or sexual understanding, paradoxically, is linked to sextimacy events and risky sexual behaviors. As Tolman describes, "Not feeling sexual desire may put girls in danger and 'at risk.' When a girl does not know what her own feelings are, when she disconnects the apprehending psychic part of herself from what is happening in her own body, she then becomes especially vulnerable to the power of others' feelings as well as to what others say she does and does not want or feel."[25]

When girls and women are out of touch with who they are, they look to others to fill in the gaps. In this way, they substitute the self of another for their own, and as such, the needs, likes, dislikes, thoughts, and feelings of others become their own. As an example of this disconnected sexuality, one adolescent girl describes a friend to Tolman: "I don't think [a friend who has a lot of sex out of relationships] knows what she wants? I think that's part of the problem . . . she's just willing to do what the people around her are doing."[26]

Many women cope and function within current constraints by not challenging the status quo and keeping others pleased with them, even when it means disconnecting from their own experiences. These messages and resulting sextimacy events may have serious long-term consequences for women with regard to love and commitment. As sextimacy events repeat, deficits develop in terms of a woman's ability to enjoy intimate sex with a monogamous partner. Studies are finding that women are more likely to be unfaithful to their spouses now than at any other time in history. Younger women (under thirty-five) are reporting more adultery than in the past, and the number of occurrences is nearly the same as that reported by men.[27]

CONCLUSION

Like a toy doll encased within a set of nesting boxes, women must pull apart layer upon layer of cultural constraints to reveal their true selves.

The messages described in this chapter are confusing, paradoxical, and in some cases oxymoronic, and as such, women who are trapped within these constraints are led to function in a similarly fragmented state. The more prone a particular woman is to seeing herself through the eyes of others, the harder it is for her to know herself through her own eyes. It may become difficult to know if a relationship is secure or risky, if a partner is trustworthy or phony, if a boyfriend is deeply loving or merely sexually intriguing. Women disconnect in order to cope with the barrage of dilemmas and inconsistencies presented to them. At the same time, disconnecting takes them further away from the happiness they seek.

The underlying reality is that many if not most women are fulfilled by authentic, real-life, trustworthy connections with other women and with men. Meeting this goal is entirely dependent on learning to accept and connect with one's self on an intimate level. In my experience treating adolescent and adult women, I find that those who maintain relationships in which their needs habitually go unmet have a depleted sense of self. At times, emotional development and self-esteem become thwarted as a result of social and family influences. When women who struggle with sextimacy become aware of how the negative thoughts and feelings they harbor about themselves originally developed, they tend to achieve greater self-acceptance. The next chapter will explore how family and social background may contribute to the occurrence of sextimacy in adulthood.

3

SUGAR, SPICE, ALL THINGS NICE

Family and Social Influence

When I learned I was pregnant with a baby boy, an old friend and mother of five told me, "Thank God, girls are such bitches!" She went on to say that her male children tended to be easy while her girls were "drama queens," always fussing and becoming emotional over seemingly inconsequential events. Another friend recalled that after bickering with her husband one morning, her four-year-old daughter asked, "Mommy, why didn't you kiss daddy goodbye?" This little girl's sharp emotional radar picked up that something was different between mommy and daddy and wanted to find out more information. Most little girls are born with an innate aptitude for reading emotional cues and for verbalizing their emotional reactions. This is a common sex difference that many parents notice early in their child's development. Nonetheless, parents and other authority figures communicate to girls and adult women that noticing and expressing emotions is a weakness. In many ways, society holds male development as the model of normal and, in turn, treats what is different as inherently wrong. All sorts of judgmental terms are used to communicate to young girls, and later to adult women, that others do not welcome their negative emotional reactions.

Parents, teachers, sports coaches, and others who impact girls on a regular basis often unintentionally use words that make them feel embarrassed and ashamed of their emotional experiences. This is so common that the words we use to judge and shame women about their emotionality are part of our everyday vernacular. Little girls may be told in various ways to put a lid on the full range of their emotions, while teenagers are called "drama queens," and adult women are told they are "needy" when they express their more negative emotional experiences. Young girls and adult women may be characterized as "high maintenance" in the sense that their emotions demand too much attention from others. And it is not only men who shame women for their emotionality; women also do this to one another.

As girls are criticized, they begin to hide the feelings they believe will be perceived negatively by others. By the time girls enter high school, many know they are not to be overly emotional and particularly not with the opposite sex. In an effort to seem more "like a guy" and less "sensitive," girls learn how to tactically mask certain emotions. At the same time, they have natural biological tendencies and social experiences that work in tandem, further reinforcing their astute emotional awareness. They experience the full spectrum of emotions and, yet, learn to hide what they feel from others so as to preserve their relationships. Without the release valve of emotional expression, many girls and women appear fine on the outside while feeling entirely emotionally depleted on the inside.

In this chapter, we explore how girls are influenced by their biology, social world, and family experience. Biology and socialization factors often interact in such a way that girls sense the complexities within their environments and relationships, yet many feel they have to hide what they are thinking and feeling. Certain family dynamics worsen these biological and social realities. When raised in family environments that do not value them on an individual basis, girls naturally have difficulty valuing themselves. This lack of self-worth leaves some particularly vulnerable to sextimacy in young adulthood. In the second half of this chapter, we will explore specific family dynamics that are associated with sextimacy.

PRIMED FOR VOICE

It is a pleasure to watch little girls when they first learn to speak, before they have any concern for the judgments of others. A friend and her two-year-old daughter, Abby, recently came over to have lunch with my son and me. Abby passionately scarfed down a chicken sandwich, demanded "MORE CHICK!" and, after loudly proclaiming "ALL DONE!", crawled into her mother's lap and unabashedly said, "I want to go home NOW, Mama." Abby was transparent; you could peer straight into the inner workings of her mind. She naturally communicated her internal voice without caution or fear about what I or her mother might think of her. Unfortunately, for girls in our culture, this is all too often a brief stage before their expanding vocabulary brushes up against constraints. Even as toddlers, little girls are beginning to tune into social cues that condition them to be above all else "nice" and keep others pleased with them.

Research on physiological brain differences in the development of language between the sexes is generally inconclusive. When differences between men and women are found, they are usually small. It seems more likely that an interaction of factors, biology, parental socialization, and society create sex differences in communication patterns. Nonetheless, there are a few differences that give girls advanced verbal ability and emotional attunement.

Girls generally learn language earlier and have more advanced language skills than boys. Compared with boys, girls have better-developed vocabularies, greater word fluency, and superior reading abilities.[1] Women who experience left-hemisphere (where language resides for most people) brain damage typically suffer fewer speech difficulties than do men with the same injury. Neurological research also demonstrates that the corpus callosum, the fiber that connects the left and right hemispheres of the brain (in particular, the area referred to as the splenium), may be larger in females.[2] As a result of this anatomical difference, women are thought to have greater hemispheric communication than men, meaning it is easier for the right hemisphere to talk with the left hemisphere.[3] For most people, emotion is processed in the right hemisphere of the brain while language resides in the left; readily integrating emotions with words is a function of both hemispheres working together. Greater ease of hemispheric communication may be a factor in girls acquiring language at a faster rate than boys, as well as their ability to more easily verbalize their emotional experiences.

Women's ability to verbalize feelings more readily than men begins at a young age. Research suggests that by age two, girls already have a more extensive emotional vocabulary than boys.[4] An interaction occurs between biology and caretakers' responses that further primes girls toward skillful internal labeling and outward verbalization of their emotional states. For example, mothers and fathers are more apt to talk with their daughters than with their sons about emotion. Parents are more likely to draw out their girls when they are in a sad mood and wonder with them about what may have caused their sadness. Parents encourage girls, more so than boys, to express the full range of human emotion (with the exception of anger, as discussed below). Mothers and fathers also tend to more positively receive their daughters' communications of feelings than they do their sons'. Likewise, both mothers and fathers tend to express their feelings to a greater extent with their daughters than they do with their sons.[5]

A natural extension of girls' astute emotional awareness and verbal aptitude is that they are prepared to orient toward relationships with others. Biology, parenting, and socialization work together, strengthening a young girl's sensitivity toward keeping others at the forefront of her mind. As infants, girls show greater attunement to their caretakers' signals and demonstrate greater empathy for their caretakers' distress than do infant boys. Girls are more likely to stay away from a new toy than are boys when their mothers appear fearful of the object. Boys are less likely to use their mothers' facial expressions to inform their behavior, and in one study, boys actually moved closer to the toy if their mothers exhibited fearful facial cues.[6]

Just as girls naturally read the emotions of others, they also feel the rewards and costs of social approval and social disapproval. Early in their development, they learn how to inhibit the expression of negative emotion if they feel it will hurt someone's feelings. For example, preschool boys are more likely than preschool girls to display a negative emotion through facial expression and behavior when receiving an undesirable gift. In an effort to not hurt the gift giver's feelings, girls tend to smile more when they receive an unwanted gift. When researchers explicitly asked boys to trick an experimenter into believing that they desired a disappointing gift, boys were unable to do this as well as girls. Taking it a step further, when researchers offered boys a prize for tricking the experimenter into believing they liked the gift, boys still were unable to suppress their negative feelings.[7]

In their development, girls learn that the expression of anger is often met with social disapproval. While mothers are often attentive to their toddler sons' expressions of anger, they tend to ignore or even inhibit their daughters' expressions of anger.[8] Just as men learn that it is more socially acceptable for them to display anger than sadness, women are conditioned to avoid the public expression of anger. Instead, women learn it is more socially acceptable to express sadness, or even distress, than anger.[9]

By the age of eight or nine, many girls are well into suppressing what they are truly thinking and feeling. Girls learn to foster their relationships by being empathic and by verbally expressing a limited range of their actual emotional perceptions. Although girls and women are acutely aware of fine distinctions in their experiences with others and themselves, many learn to communicate only that which shows attentiveness to the feelings of others. And so it goes that the natural gifts young girls have to voice their experiences may become deeply buried.

THE BIND

In order to maintain the self-esteem they take from their relationships, girls and adult women may subvert their thoughts and feelings to keep others happy with them. This bind is thoughtfully described in Mary Pipher's deeply insightful book, *Reviving Ophelia.* Pipher outlines how society places young girls in an impossible dilemma, namely that they are to display feminine traits, such as selflessness, demureness, and a commitment to making relationships work. On the other hand, they have a separate set of natural needs and opinions that do not always match the expectations thrust upon them.[10] It is not unusual for adolescent girls and young women to feel they must hide their true selves from others.

Adolescent girls make telling sacrifices in authenticity and relinquish parts of themselves in order to connect with and keep others close.[11] Girls and women often feel forced to give up stating what they are truly feeling and thinking so that they may be pleasing to others and maintain closeness. This hyper-focus on relationships thwarts a girl's quest to develop her own identity separate from how she experiences herself in a relationship.

This learning begins early when many girls discover that relationships with caregivers run more smoothly when they do not express negative emotion and, as a result, begin to turn down the volume on their emotional worlds. Based on the ability to be intimately in tune with changes in her environment and the emotions of others, a little girl may be quite perceptive at noticing her mother's sadness or anger. And she may have little difficulty labeling her own negative emotions. However, if caregivers treat emotional expression dismissively, or even angrily, girls perceive that it is unacceptable to talk about the negative emotions that they are noticing or feeling. This learning history sets the stage for the young girl to stifle her negative experiences with others and adopt an inauthentic self that conforms to the expectations of others.

So what are these girls to do? They feel everything. They are masterfully skillful at reading and understanding emotion, and relationships are their primary source of happiness and self-esteem. Concurrently, girls are often indirectly told that in order to preserve their relationships, they are to be pleasing to others and only communicate positive or neutral emotion. These messages are fundamentally in opposition and encourage the development of a false self. Those in this dilemma internalize their feelings, repetitively replay upsetting emotional events in their minds, use drama as an emotional outlet, and influence their relationships through indirect aggression. These coping mechanisms are ineffective and deplete a woman's emotional health.

REPETITIVE THINKING

Without the option of safe, direct, emotional expression within their intimate relationships, there is no release valve for young women, and their negative experiences are internalized. Girls frequently report to me that they are caught in an overthinking trap and wish they could turn off their minds. They are panicked about keeping their relationships intact, and so they are indirect with others about their needs or about their more negative emotional experiences. Instead, they try to problem solve the upset internally through repetitively replaying negative events in their minds and constantly second-guessing themselves.

They tell themselves in many different ways that they should not feel whatever negative emotion they are, in fact, experiencing. They tell themselves, "Why am I upset? This really isn't a big deal . . . What is wrong with me that I am upset all of the time? . . . All I do is feel sorry for myself . . . I am so selfish to be angry . . . Why am I so sensitive?", and the list continues. If relationships are a primary source of self-esteem for girls and women, then communicating negative emotions to others is equivalent to biting the hand that feeds you. For some, it feels too threatening to be emotionally real because, in their view, openly expressing negative emotion places relationships at risk.

In psychology literature, the tendency to repeat and work through negative events in one's mind is termed *rumination.* Rumination refers to internally focusing on upset or distress, as well as all of the reasons, causes, future possibilities, or risks that could occur due to this distress. An example might be sitting alone, thinking about feeling lonely and worrying that there will never be anyone, then imagining a future of aloneness and focusing on all the perceived things that caused this state of aloneness. Rumination is a passive, helpless process, and girls and women are more likely than boys and men to self-report that they overthink when feeling distressed.[12] Whereas men can become more easily distracted from their sad mood or externalize their feelings, women tend to ruminate and mentally replay upsetting events.[13]

Depression is more prevalent among women than men. This is a solid research finding in epidemiology, one that has been extensively researched and culturally cross-validated.[14] Women begin to have higher rates of depression than men in early adolescence, and this trend continues throughout their development. Interestingly, the adolescent period is when relationships start to become more complex, and this is when young women start ruminating more. Rumination is inherently tied to depression; the more a woman ruminates, the more likely she is to become depressed. Many researchers believe rumination explains women's increased risk for depression.

Although women often tell me that rumination feels productive in the moment, like they are problem solving, it ultimately prolongs their distress and depletes their mood. Squelching the expression of negative emotion results in rumination and depression, as well as acute feelings of powerlessness and worthlessness.[15] In some ways, rumination is a way to privately keep one's voice alive—to keep alive what the self knows to be true but cannot express. Nonetheless, rumination is a poor substitute for authentic connection and taking direct action in relationships.

RELATIONAL AGGRESSION

Researchers have identified that like boys, girls are aggressive but are more likely to engage in indirect or relational aggression.[16] Examples of relational aggression include punishing a friend by excluding her from her primary social group, ignoring a friend, not inviting a friend to a special party, ostracizing a close friend, ganging up as a group on one rejected member, name calling, and giving dirty looks and mean stares. These are ways to assert the negative emotion one might feel about another without having to directly confront the person. Girls (and even some adult women) are more likely than boys and men to engage in relational aggression or female bullying.

Girls and women know that relationships are primary for one another, and when they are unable to manage their needs or negative emotions directly, they use relationships as a weapon. In my work with young women, there are two relationally aggressive dynamics that are the most depleting to girls and women's sense of self and wellbeing. The first is when the social group suddenly turns against one member and stops speaking to or including her in the social circle. The second is when one member of the clique becomes the subject of gossip. Rather than directly speaking to the girl in question, one member begins to talk about her to others in the clique and may spread rumors to those outside of the clique.

Girls and women place high value on their relationships. They become painfully self-critical when they feel unwanted by others.[17] For many girls, their self-esteem rests on their ability to stay connected with others. When they feel unwanted and are given no direct reason as to why, girls and women often feel rejected and worthless. Girls become emotionally overwhelmed by bullying and are so caught up in self-blame that they have trouble organizing or making sense of their reactions. Feeling emotionally overwhelmed often becomes misinterpreted as "drama," a highly judgmental label that further renders young girls and adult women fearful of expressing their more negative emotions or experiences.

DRAMA

There can be roadblocks in social relationships that prevent girls from effectively expressing their true selves. As a result, they may turn to repetitive thinking and/or indirect aggression. At some point, these tactics stop working, and intense emotion comes flooding in. The intense expression of emotion by girls and young women may be labeled drama. The women and girls I see who tend toward drama are those who have difficulty understanding and expressing their emotional experiences on an ongoing basis.

The word *drama* reflects the training girls receive early in their development that says they are not to burden others with their intense, emotional reactions. Calling drama on another girl suggests that whatever she is experiencing is somehow false or is being expressed to achieve an unrealistic need or ulterior motive. People do not trust drama, and many girls and women work to not express what they are feeling lest they be branded a needy drama queen. The interesting paradox is that the more you manage emotions through actively pushing them away, the more intense they become. Emotions want airtime and need to be attended to and validated. Emotions resist attempts to be stifled, and drama is typically the result of this stifling (as will be discussed in chapter 4). Hiding feelings and repressing negative experiences eventually give way, and the women involved become emotionally overwhelmed.

Women are often accused of being overly emotional; in my experience, they actually spend a great deal of time talking themselves out of their emotional reactions or judging themselves harshly for what they feel. Those who are better able to validate their emotional experiences and manage to find direct outlets for such are less likely to have overwhelming emotional episodes. As we have seen, understanding and directly expressing emotion on a day-to-day basis is extremely difficult for some because they perceive it may lead to conflict and the loss of a relationship. An example of drama is seen in the story of Kim.

Kim, a seventeen-year-old senior in high school, entered psychotherapy for anxiety. She felt constantly nervous, excluded and disliked by her friends. When she came to see me, she was caught in a repetitive thinking trap. She continually told herself that she was overly sensitive for feeling hurt and disappointed in her relationships. For her first three years in high school, Kim led her social clique and felt liked and accepted. When we explored why she was now feeling anxious about her friends, she listed numerous instances where she felt they betrayed her trust. She described her best friend telling others in her social group that Kim acted like a "slut." Sometimes she was invited on outings with her group, and other times she heard about their fun after the fact. She felt intimate secrets she shared in confidence, with a select few, were now being scattered about the school. In spite of this, Kim was clear about one thing: She wanted to stay connected with her social clique and eventually return to her full status as an integral member.

Kim continued to feel left out and mistreated by her friends, but she believed this was the currency she had to pay in order to work her way back into the group. After enduring hurt again and again, Kim was at the end of her rope. While drinking with friends at a party, she was startled to realize her best friend had disappeared. Concerned, she began to search the house and discovered her best friend hooking up. The hookup was with Kim's former boyfriend. Kim held in her distress about so many things and for so long that it was like a dam breaking. Kim became angry. While fellow partygoers gawked, she screamed at her friend and then broke down crying. After the event, Kim was humiliated—mortified that she let her guard down. When she returned to school, she heard others from the party saying things like, "Here comes drama" when she walked down the hall. This event confirmed Kim's belief that it was unacceptable to express negative emotions. She went back to settling for whatever leftovers her social group would give her, became coy and quiet about her upset, and conformed to whatever the larger group wanted from her. In order to preserve her relationships, Kim learned to adopt an inauthentic self.

While in therapy, Kim came to understand the valid and justifiable reasons for the negative emotions she experienced. She had been repeatedly mistreated, yet told herself that it was her fault that she felt hurt. She continued to put herself in the line of fire, essentially agreeing to be walked on by her friends. The upset and distress she experienced went unattended and, as such, ballooned out of proportion. It was actually a healthy sign that Kim eventually allowed herself to feel her emotions and become angry with her peer group. Once she began to pay attention to the negative things that happened to her, Kim no longer put herself in harm's way and stopped tolerating mistreatment in her relationships.

PATTERNS IN FAMILIES

Certain family backgrounds set the stage for girls to engage in repetitive thinking, relational aggression, and drama and condition girls toward one-sided relationships in adulthood. There are three family dynamics that are common in the backgrounds of girls and women who struggle with sextimacy: the parental pop-in, a lack of boundaries, and the invalidating parent/child relationship. You may find that one of these family patterns matches your own background, or you may relate to a combination of these. These dynamics are often played out repeatedly by women in their adult relationships with men. As you read through the next section, consider the dynamic(s) that may apply to you. In chapter 7, we will explore how these and other love patterns can be altered through challenging one's self to engage new types of romantic partners.

The Parental Pop-In

The parental pop-in is a dynamic whereby one parent only shows up for the fun but is absent for the day-to-day grind of life. The children in such an environment feel unknown by the pop-in parent and, therefore, work hard to always be on their best behavior whenever in the presence of this parent. A young girl in such an environment may feel disappointed that her parent is not around consistently and simultaneously guilty for harboring upset with the parent. She learns to repress these feelings.

An example of the pop-in is seen in the story of Stephanie. Stephanie grew up in an environment where, although her parents were married, they lived separate lives. Stephanie was quite close to her mother and openly shared the intimacies of day-to-day life with her. She did not see her father as often, but when she did, it was typically fun and stress free. She recalled one story when she was seven, and her father had been on a business trip for a few weeks. It was her birthday, and she felt panic that he might not be back in time for her big day. On her birthday, Stephanie went to school feeling a bit disappointed that he was not home yet. Just as her teacher was beginning the day's lesson, a school official entered the classroom with twelve red roses and three big balloons. She could hardly believe that she was receiving these gifts at school and felt special when the teacher tied the balloons to her desk chair. She felt like a princess all day and was beyond excited to go home and celebrate with both of her parents.

Only when she arrived home, her father was not there. Stephanie's mother conveyed that he was unable to make it home until the next day. She felt crushed. The adrenaline and excitement she felt about the balloons and her birthday gave way to tears and sadness. Stephanie's mother tried to console her through unveiling her birthday gift, a new puppy. Although she was pleased with the puppy, what Stephanie really wanted was her father's presence. She felt guilty expressing this because, after all, he had done so much for her.

Through the years, this theme continued. When Stephanie's father returned from a business trip, he would often do something spontaneous and grand for the family. Stephanie described numerous lush and exciting family vacations, where her father was always jovial and generous. He would even bring up things that he wanted to do with Stephanie when the family returned home. He would promise to attend her next soccer game or take her to school. Each time Stephanie was left deflated and disappointed because her father never delivered the attention he promised and that she so sorely craved. As time passed, Stephanie became increasingly skilled at suppressing her disappointment and telling herself that her father was doing everything for her, so how could she have anything but positive feelings toward him?

Stephanie's story illustrates the dynamic of a parent who pops in bringing joy and pops out leaving a wake of sadness. Young children have a tendency to be egocentric in their thinking. It is hard for them to grasp the complexities of other people's perspectives and motives. This egocentric thinking means they believe, on some level, that they both cause the pop-in and cause the pop-out. They work diligently to be good enough so that they may always keep the parent as close as possible. Of course they are not responsible for the pop-in or pop-out and have no real control over its occurrence. Nonetheless, the child is left feeling that her best is not good enough and senses she cannot predict or create her own happiness.

There are two other consequences to the parental pop-in that influence adult relationships and sextimacy events: invalidation and lack of intimacy. Because caregivers never took her disappointment and hurt seriously, the child tends to invalidate her emotional experiences in relationships. Early on, she learns to tell herself that everything is fine, even when she knows on a deeper level that she is far from fine. This learning history sets the stage for her to repeat this family dynamic in her adult romantic relationships. When she is mistreated or disappointed by a guy who is not attending to her needs, she easily tells herself, "It's no big deal, get over it." In addition, the pop-in parent does not know the child on an intimate and day-to-day level. This means the child only knows how to share what she perceives as the more acceptable parts of herself with those she loves most.

The parental pop-in manifests in adult relationships where an individual feels unknown by the person with whom she is romantically involved. Like her childhood relationships, she engages in adult relationships that are inconsistent, leaving her to feel higher than a kite at times and lower than low at others—and, of course, this is how a sextimacy event feels.

No Boundaries

Parents who do not provide adequate boundaries expose their daughters to adulthood before they are cognitively prepared. Parent/child boundaries may be blurred and even crossed in a variety of ways, including chronically exposing children to parental conflict, inviting children into parental conflict, using the child as a bargaining chip, as well as exposing children to parental sexual activity. Children are naturally curious about their parents' relationship, and girls, in particular, are quite aware of emotional currents within the family. Girls will ask questions about their parents, and it is the parents' job to protect their children from harsher adult realities until they are more mature. Healthy parents will argue in front of their children, as this helps children to see how conflict is managed and demonstrates that people who love one another can respectfully disagree. When boundaries are missing, however, arguments may turn into knock-down, drag-out assaults with personal cruelty on full display. This is harmful for the child because it can feel as if the assault is happening to her.

Many young girls feel every emotion that their parents experience during a fight—anger, hurt, defensiveness, physiological arousal—yet, unlike their parents, young girls do not have the emotional maturity to understand what they are feeling, much less to protect themselves from the barrage. Chronic parental conflict and unhappiness often results in a parent confiding in a daughter as a way to gain emotional comfort. For example, some mothers openly discuss their marital conflict with their daughters, and some even discuss their sex lives. Discussing private details of marital life creates an atmosphere that is emotionally confusing for the child, who is cognitively and emotionally unprepared to manage such matters. It leaves the child once again in a relationship that is more about the needs of the other than herself.

Another way that boundaries become blurred is in the case of divorce and separation. When divorce or separation occurs, many parents begin to more openly discuss and display the conflicts within their marriage to their children. As they are typically emotionally overwhelmed themselves, parents in a disintegrating marriage tend to become self-focused and are more apt to fight in front of their children. Parents often regress during marital separation and may act in an adolescent manner. This is a particularly harmful boundary violation when the children involved are adolescents themselves. A daughter has a sudden loss of innocence if a parent begins dating quickly or discussing his or her sex life. The child is abruptly thrust into the adult world of relationships. She comes to understand things like infidelity, jealousy, and cheating, and this provides her with a cynical and untrusting perception of relationships and men. As the parent engages in dating and sex, these acts become normalized to the adolescent, compressing the time they wait to have sex or hook up. Jamie is an example of how this can play out.

Until she was eleven, Jamie lived a fairly safe and easy life. She believed her parents loved each other and never even considered that life could change, or that they would turn mean and ugly toward one another. Knowing she had a solid family foundation, Jamie felt secure and focused on her own life. Suddenly and seemingly out of nowhere, events changed. Her mother came home one day distraught. She frantically searched through drawers and closets; she was throwing things and crying. Jamie felt pained and terrified to see her mother in such a state. Jamie asked what was going on, and her mother angrily said, "You want to know what is going on? Your father is cheating, that is what is going on!" Jamie was confused about the meaning of this statement and initially thought it meant that her father was somehow copying someone else's answers at work. Her mother used words that were overwhelming for Jamie, words that she had never before paired with her father: jealousy, liar, cheat, hypocrite, deceptive, untrustworthy. Jamie felt her heart race. Her face became hot. She had no words to describe what she felt.

Years later in therapy, Jamie reflected on this experience and said it was as if her foundation disappeared, leaving her in free fall. This flood of emotion and harsh language permanently altered Jamie's reality. She no longer felt safe or secure. She turned her attention to comforting her mother. As the weeks passed, her parents fought on a constant basis; often the argument culminated in one or the other leaving the house in a rage. Eventually, her father left the family home for good, and Jamie's mother immediately began dating. Boyfriends were in the home regularly. She shared with Jamie information about the men she found attractive, identified those who were better lovers than her father, and explained her need to "play hard to get" with those she dated. By the time Jamie entered high school, she knew more about cheating, infidelity, and playing the game with men than many adults. She had developed a jaded view of men, and felt it was unlikely that any man could be trustworthy and giving toward her. In addition, when she arrived home from school each day, she listened to her mother talk either about her heartbreak or her dating life.

Jamie no longer had the foundation of a caring family and, instead, entered a world where her emotional needs were neglected for the needs of others. She was left with a depleted self, a belief that her needs would not be attended to in relationships, and a distorted view of men and their ability to be trustworthy. Experiencing a lack of parental boundaries as a child manifests in adult romantic relationships where needs go habitually unmet, and a tendency develops toward dating or hooking up with immature men. These are blocks to emotional intimacy and are antithetical to long-term, secure relationships.

Parental Invalidation

Parental invalidation is a way that some parents limit a daughter's negative and emotional expressions in the household. Paradoxically, the invalidating family begets greater emotionality because the young girl is given no guidance to understand and manage her emotional world. Parental invalidation threatens a girl's prospects for developing a healthy, nondepleted sense of self.

This family climate is characterized by indirectly or directly telling girls that they do not, should not, or cannot feel something that they do, in fact, truly feel. An example of the direct invalidation is seen in a mother whose child keeps saying, "I am hungry," and the mother replies, "No, you're not hungry, you're fine." Less direct invalidation is seen by parents who, when faced with their child's upset, respond dismissively: "Why are you feeling sorry for yourself? . . . There is nothing to be upset about . . . Think positively." As these trivializing phrases accumulate, they communicate to a young girl that she should not be feeling what she is feeling. This is a confusing message, and the young girl who receives it begins to conclude that she is somehow misperceiving reality. Invalidation communicates to girls that their needs and negative emotional states are a burden to others.

In no time at all, a girl with an invalidating family background may become conditioned to be quite careful about what she expresses. She may feel ashamed of herself when, in a weak moment, she expresses negative emotions. By the time these girls enter high school, many are so accustomed to invalidating themselves that they enter therapy believing there is something wrong with them for feeling negative emotion. They tell me all of the reasons they should not be feeling the things they really are feeling and want help from me to not feel these things. They have tremendous difficulty actually speaking openly about what ails them.

While girls in invalidating families are being criticized for expressing their emotions, they are often used simultaneously as emotional receptacles by caregivers and friends. This is a double whammy. Their emotional astuteness makes them easy to talk to, and as a result, some parents unwittingly lean on them for their own invalidated emotional needs. So, for these girls, their personal emotions are unacceptable for others to know, but they are expected to be caring and giving when others wish to emote.

The invalidating environment conditions the young girl to believe that sharing her emotions is not safe, as she will invariably be made to feel worse about herself in some way. As a consequence, she feels uncared for and unseen, unless she is in the service of someone else's needs. This environment sets the stage for the development of one-sided romantic relationships in adulthood, where her needs are less attended to than those of the other. An example of parental invalidation is seen in the story of Melanie.

Melanie, a twenty-year-old college student, came to therapy wrought with anxiety and depression. She was struggling with sextimacy events and feeling worthless because she was unable to manage a committed relationship. While growing up, her parents were divorced, and she spent most of her time with her mother. Melanie, an emotionally aware eight-year-old at the time of her parents' divorce, began to use her emotional astuteness to make her mother happy. Melanie described trying to cheer up her mother with songs and dances and even watching grownup television shows to keep her mother company. Melanie felt attached to her mother and wanted to ensure her happiness. Because of her concern for her mother, Melanie did not focus on her own feelings about the divorce. As she reflected on her parents' divorce in therapy, she was unable to recall anyone asking her how she felt about her father leaving and divorcing her mother.

Melanie did recall becoming overwhelmed by an intense bout of sadness soon after her father left her family home and turning to her mother for support. Melanie's mother, herself emotionally overwhelmed, responded in a dismissive way, "Why are you crying, everything is fine in your world, life is so easy for you," or "You have nothing to feel upset about, you will still see your father, but me, I am alone forever."

As an adult, Melanie described that, on the one hand, she had a very close relationship with her mother, while on the other hand, she was unable to talk with her mother about her more complicated emotional self. In a weak moment, Melanie might call her mother and share her upset, hoping that her mother would finally get it. Invariably, Melanie's mother would respond with the same kind of dismissive comments she used when Melanie was a child: "Nothing's really wrong . . . Why are you feeling sorry for yourself? . . . Look at all I have done for you . . . You're pretty, you have friends, you have a great life, what is there to be upset about?"

As an adult, Melanie chose friends and boyfriends who invalidated her emotions just as her mother did. Therapy helped Melanie learn to validate her feelings, take her needs seriously, and become more direct with people about her goals. This helped Melanie become more comfortable with herself and to develop romantic relationships with partners who attended to her emotional needs.

The invalidating environment sets the stage for women to believe that it is actually weak, shameful, and burdensome to share their negative emotions with others. They may pride themselves on not having to be "needy" and rarely let their guard down to reveal the real pain they experience. Not only do they have pain as adults that they mask, but they also have years of unaddressed childhood pain. Adult women raised in an invalidating environment are left with missing data about themselves and feel a great deal of confusion about who they really are. They also have tremendous difficulty understanding or organizing their emotional experiences, and emotions quickly become heated and intense.

When the invalidating family background does not become adequately processed and understood, adult relationships are difficult to develop, and the women involved begin to believe that they will never find a partner with whom they can be candid. Most importantly, it is hard for these women to not only get close to others, but also to let others get close to them. Although they crave unconditional acceptance, they fear revealing their shortcomings and keep communication on a surface level.

SEXTIMACY LINK

Most girls are born with well-tuned emotional radar and a compassionate desire to support and nurture others. They also experience emotional ups and downs, disappointments and heartbreaks. The contradiction between what girls and women really are versus what many are trained to believe they should be creates emotional turmoil and a depleted self.

The old nursery rhyme is catchy, but little girls are made up of a whole lot more than sugar and spice and all things nice. The notion that girls should be nice and sweet is often communicated by well-meaning parents and caregivers who may not recognize the stifling and restrictive messages they are sending. The consequence can be profound: Girls and women become limited in their experience and understanding of themselves. This keep-a-lid-on-it attitude makes girls, and later women, unready to effectively manage their emotional experiences. Girls become accustomed to one-sided relationships where they dismiss their own needs.

All of the training a girl receives in one-sided relationships becomes reenacted within her romantic relationships. Although she may feel miserable after a sextimacy event, she tells herself that "everything is fine" and "there is nothing to be upset about." She sacrifices what she knows to be true in order to maintain the relationship. Before picking a sextimacy partner, she may sense problems about the man but, again, dismisses her feelings and pushes forth. Like the parental pop-in, she subsists on the good times in the relationship and denies the disappointment she experiences for the better part of the liaison. She is well trained in settling for inconsistent attention, and this perpetuates the sextimacy cycle.

CONCLUSION

Many girls learn through their social and family experiences to silence their inner voices, preparing them to settle for one-sided relationships in adulthood. Treating adolescent and adult women, I find that those who maintain relationships in which their needs habitually go unmet have specific areas of self that are not fully developed. The next three chapters are directed toward helping those in this situation develop a strong self-identity by effectively understanding and managing their emotional world, improving their ability to directly communicate, and building self-esteem. As a woman develops a strong core sense of self, fulfilling relationships where her needs are consistently met will follow. By developing in this way, women are less vulnerable to sextimacy and more able to get what they truly want from men—authentic connection, sexual fulfillment, and emotional intimacy.

SELF-ASSESSMENT: ARE YOU AT RISK FOR ONE-SIDED ROMANTIC RELATIONSHIPS?

After reading about the social and cultural factors involved in sextimacy, you may be wondering if your background places you at risk for one-sided, sextimacy relationships. Take this self-assessment to assess your level of risk; the more items you endorse, the more vulnerable you are to sextimacy.

1. Are you intuitive and instinctively sense what others may be feeling?
2. Do you have a great deal of empathy and easily feel others' suffering as if it were your own?
3. Do you easily know if someone's mood is off or if they are having a hard day, even if they do not directly communicate this to you?
4. Do your friends turn to you for emotional support, and then when you need someone, do you feel there is no one for you to go to?
5. Do you have trouble opening up to others on a regular basis and then suddenly have an emotional explosion?
6. When you become upset, do you find that it is very hard to calm down?
7. Do you tell yourself that you should not be feeling something you are feeling?
8. Do you judge yourself harshly when you have an emotional outburst?
9. When you were a child, would your parents not ask you to elaborate about how your school day went?
10. Were either of your parents prone to great emotionality—anxiety attacks, depressive bouts, episodes of rage/anger?
11. Looking back, is it hard to remember one of your parents comforting you when you were upset?
12. Were your parents unlikely to take responsibility if they hurt your feelings, and did they fail to say things like, "I am sorry that happened. I can understand why you would feel that way."
13. Did you know about sex earlier than your peers?
14. Did either of your parents openly date others in a way that made you feel uncomfortable or have affairs that you knew about?
15. Did either of your parents discuss their own sex life or casually allow you to find condoms, overhear them on a phone with a lover, or watch them flirt with strangers?
16. When upset, do you tend to overthink or repetitively replay events in your mind without getting anywhere?

17. Do you have difficulty being direct with friends or romantic partners about what you want or need in the relationship?
18. Did you feel you had to always keep up a good mood or be positive when you were around one of your parents?
19. Do you feel unknown by many of your friends and family members?
20. Did you have intercourse or engage in oral sex before the age of sixteen?

4

Drama

Developing Emotional Awareness

At eleven months, Emily was an emotionally exuberant little girl. She wore her emotions on her sleeve; no one smiled bigger when filled with joy or cried harder with disappointment. She felt everything and was vibrantly alive. Her parents were often exasperated by Emily's emotional energy because when she was upset, it was hard to make her feel better. On one occasion, Emily was ready for a nap when her older brother snatched away her favorite toy doll. He threw it up on a shelf that Emily could not reach. Emily was frustrated and angry and began to wail. She cried so hard, she reached a point where she could not breathe. Her little mouth was open, but without breath, there was no sound. She fainted.

Emily's parents were terrified. They believed her life was in danger. They rushed Emily to an emergency room, but during the car ride to the hospital she regained consciousness and was calm. The doctor who examined Emily dismissed the incident, chuckling to Emily's parents, "Looks like you've got a breath holder here: a little drama queen in the making." Emily's parents were relieved that she was safe, and it felt good to laugh about the whole ordeal. However, this incident profoundly impacted the ways in which Emily's parents responded to her emotions and eventually set the stage for how Emily responded to herself emotionally.

Emily's doctor did not explain to her parents that she suffered what is medically termed a "breath-holding spell," a brief period when a young child may stop breathing or pass out due to intense emotion. The intense emotion causes a change in the child's heart rate and ability to take a breath, thus causing the child to faint. Breath-holding spells are reflexive, automatic, and most importantly, they are no more likely to occur in female children than in male children.[1]

Armed with the illuminating label *drama queen*, Emily's parents felt empowered. A medical expert confirmed what they had suspected. They began to treat Emily differently. They were no longer empathetic in response to emotional outbursts; after all, Emily's problem was too much drama. Emily's parents insidiously began to dismiss her emotional reactions. Every time Emily would cry or have trouble transitioning from one activity to another, her parents would respond with something like, "You have to buck up . . . Big girls don't cry . . . Mommy can't take your crying anymore." Through the years, Emily's parents felt the only way to break Emily of her dramatic episodes was not to play into her "manipulations for attention" and chose to isolate Emily when she became upset. They would put her in her room, shut the door, and let her calm down on her own.

All of these tactics, unfortunately, had the reverse effect and left Emily completely overwhelmed and baffled by her emotional world. She developed an association between her reactions and people leaving or abandoning her. She came to believe that she was too much for people, and that if anyone knew the real her, they would not love her or want to be her friend. As the years passed, she learned to suppress, or push away, her natural emotional reactions. When speaking with her parents or her brother, she would act happy and pleased, even when something was eating her up inside. Later, she developed friendships where she prided herself on not upsetting others and never having an argument with a friend. As a result of dismissing her own feelings, Emily was left with a limited sense of who she really was and concentrated on working hard to be who she believed everyone else wanted her to be.

Repressed emotions are similar to steam in a pressure cooker demanding release. Because she could not directly express her feelings, eventually even to herself, let alone to others, Emily's feelings found other more destructive outlets. By high school, Emily was obsessively critiquing her physical appearance. She began to have panic attacks, and most distressing of all, she began cutting herself to achieve emotional relief. If negative emotion did break through her defenses, she would judge herself: "Why are you feeling this way, what is wrong with you? . . . You are you so dramatic, get a grip!"

Emily's struggles intensified once she entered college and relationships with men and women became more complex. Increasingly, Emily was unable to be alone. She surrounded herself with other people, yet at the same time, she felt lonely and unknown. Emily never knew what she felt about someone or something in the moment and was blindsided by waves of emotion after the fact. She often engaged in risky behaviors, unfulfilling sexual relationships, and one-sided friendships. She pleased others through appearing easygoing and happy. When alone, she found herself choking back tears and judging herself for feeling sad. Frightened she would be abandoned, she worked extra hard to never show the men in her life her true feelings.

This story illustrates a type of emotional learning that is actually quite common for girls in our culture. When parents do not understand themselves emotionally and have difficulty regulating their own emotions, they tend to treat their daughters' emotional sensitivity dismissively and with criticism. Although parents are usually working with the best of intentions and want to help their daughters to be strong and not thrown by life's setbacks, emotional dismissal and avoidance create a weak and fragile sense of self.

The label *drama queen* is a misnomer to the extent that it is used to mean that a woman is extremely emotional and that this is the source of all her difficulties. Actually, as mentioned earlier, quite the opposite is true; these women have been conditioned to suppress and hold back what they feel in an effort to please. Wanting to be liked and pleasing to the exclusion of understanding one's own emotional reactions perpetuates the sextimacy cycle. Developing emotional awareness is a key component to making healthy romantic choices.

THE MAKINGS OF A DRAMA QUEEN

In many cases, caregivers are emotionally ill-equipped themselves and have learned to push away their own negative emotional reactions.

They are overwhelmed when a little girl suddenly starts spouting off about her own emotions. In order to effectively help girls manage their emotional experiences, caregivers need empathy and emotional attunement; without this, they are at a loss in terms of understanding their daughters' emotional reactions.

One way that caregivers tame a girl's emotional world is through using moralistic and judgmental language that plays into her innate need to stay connected to others. In an effort not to create conflict within their relationships, girls become conditioned to tell themselves certain things when they sense an emotion coming on—"People will think I am weak if I cry again . . . I have so much to be grateful for, why do I feel this way? . . . No one will want to be around me if I am upset . . . Good girls don't get angry . . . If I tell her how I feel, that makes me a bad person because it will hurt her feelings." This type of emotional conditioning works effectively, as girls learn to have an aversion to drama and tend to judge themselves, and other girls, harshly when emotions flood in.

By the time they are young adults, many women are schooled in the art of suppressing their emotions. As a result, they may have difficulty being emotionally available or empathic to the struggles of others. They may criticize or make fun of girls or women who cry and believe they are stronger because they do not do so, at least publicly. If overly expressive about their negative emotions or upset, they call "drama" on one another. These girls and women work diligently to minimize the impact of their emotions and, at times, operate by avoiding their emotional reactions altogether and dismissing those of others.

Even girls and women who are trained to suppress emotion continue to feel emotion; it is part of the human condition. When the protective dam collapses, they are surprised by overwhelming emotion that may present itself in terms of a dramatic symptom. Symptoms of tuning out emotions include obsessing over seemingly minor events or perceived physical flaws, anxiety disorders, constant rumination, fixating on one thought (for example, worrying that a romantic relationship will end), eating disorders, cutting behaviors, or repeatedly engaging in dysfunctional dynamics in relationships with men and women.

Drama or maladaptive emotional symptoms occur when a person habitually suppresses or avoids his or her emotional experiences. Suppression works in a variety of ways depending on the individual. It may mean avoiding emotion altogether, pushing away the emotion already experienced, or judging oneself for having emotions at all. When people do not allow themselves to recognize and consider whatever it is they truly feel, they avoid the underlying condition that is the source of their pain. When this happens, negative emotion becomes channeled into some form of self-abuse.

An excellent example of self-abuse taking the place of a genuine emotional experience is the woman who, after suffering a difficult breakup, says to herself, "I am going to lose ten pounds, and that will show him." The loss, sadness, and betrayal of the breakup are blocked out by an obsessive focus on weight. When feelings get shunted to the external and remain unprocessed, internal suffering continues.

Suppression also occurs when a woman feels something but works really hard not to let others know what she is feeling. This involves inhibiting body language and verbal communication so as to conceal feelings from others. An example of this inhibition is the girlfriend or wife who is completely shocked and angry by her partner's mistreatment of her. Rather than expressing these feelings and drawing a boundary with her partner, she suppresses and focuses on his feelings so that he will not become angrier with her.

Research consistently demonstrates that suppressing emotional reactions actually intensifies negative experiences, increases the odds of having a lack of social support, and intensifies depressive symptoms.[2] One study asked depressed college students to either suppress or not suppress their negative or positive thoughts. Researchers found that those students who worked to suppress their negative thoughts actually had more negative thoughts. Essentially, when we suppress thoughts or emotional states, we tell ourselves to "stop thinking about that." The mind then begins to monitor itself for each time it does think about "that" and then brings "that" to our conscious awareness.[3]

As we will see in the next section, by the time people become conscious of what they may be feeling and work to inhibit that feeling, their brains are already engaged in a full physiological reaction. The horse is out of the barn. It takes a great deal of cognitive energy to inhibit the emotion.

Actively inhibiting an emotional experience so that others do not know what you are feeling leads to less emotional intimacy and weaker interpersonal functioning with others.[4] This is interesting to consider because women often report that they suppress their emotions in an effort to remain nice, calm, or empathic to preserve their relationships. When emotions are sharply inhibited and neither labeled nor addressed in the moment, they eventually resurface in different ways—panic attacks, passive aggressive behavior, compulsive working, obsessive thinking, compulsive eating, obsessive dieting. These symptoms may be shameful for people to talk about and may eliminate honest communication in their relationships.

To begin exploring underlying emotions, it is important to recognize that they are a natural biological function. Emotions are generated on a physiological level long before conscious awareness. Emotions are evolutionarily adaptive and serve as a guide for self-protection.[5]

WHY DO WE FEEL?

In describing his own episodes of depression, Charles Darwin wrote that sorrow "leads an animal to pursue that course of action which is most beneficial." Andy Thomson, a psychiatrist at the University of Virginia who studies evolutionary psychology, has developed the analytic-rumination hypothesis to explain the evolutionary roots of depression.[6] This theory postulates that feeling down has some evolutionary advantage as it signals the mind and body when a dilemma needs to be solved. Life becomes more productive as the self analyzes problems and conducts a cost-benefit review of the optimal way to solve a particular issue. Sadness is often accompanied by isolation and loneliness, which may increase an individual's appreciation and motivation for intimacy and closeness with others.

Every emotion is a signal about what to do in a particular situation or with a particular person. At one extreme, fear may trigger the body's fight-or-flight response. Worrying is a way to anticipate threats so they may be prevented. The experience of shame and guilt preserves certain community standards and helps individuals behave in ways that maintain social order. The brain works in a way that allows these emotional instincts to engage as needed, encouraging a person to tune in and effectively manage their circumstances.

The human brain has evolved over a vast stretch of time, but some parts are less evolved than others. The emotional centers of the brain, or limbic areas, in particular, appeared in animals hundreds of millions of years ago, developing from an even more primitive region of the brain, the brainstem. The neocortex, the area of the brain that separates humans from animals and is involved in conscious thinking, probably evolved a few million years ago and thus has had far less time to develop than the emotional areas.[7] Perhaps as a result of this evolutionary lag, connections from the emotional centers to the cognitive areas are considerably stronger than connections from the cognitive to the emotional.[8] In other words, emotion has more influence on our conscious thinking than our thinking has on emotion.

The amygdala, an almond-shaped structure located just above the brainstem, is strongly associated with emotional responses, as well as with emotional memory. This small structure gives the events and people in our lives meaning. The amygdala processes the information and decides if it is emotionally significant. Certain emotionally expressive reactions will occur throughout the body including hormonal changes, changes in heartbeat or body temperature, and muscle-tension differences. Once the emotional information enters the cortex, it can be considered thoughtfully, processed, labeled, and put into perspective.

Joseph LeDoux, a neuroscientist at the Center for Neural Science at New York University, has extensively researched the role of the amygdala in emotional processing. In his studies, he brilliantly uncovered a faster "back alley" pathway to the amygdala.[9] This separate, previously unknown pathway leads directly from the thalamus to the amygdala, skipping the cortex altogether.

This means some emotional data from the environment enter directly into the amygdala, thus giving the cortex no data about what is being processed. LeDoux found the amygdala could signal an emotional response in the brain without a person having any conscious awareness of why. Because this direct amygdala pathway is shorter, and thus faster, than the longer and more intricate pathway to the cortex, it represents an evolutionary advantage. The direct amygdala pathway allows for quick emotional processing so as to achieve an almost instantaneous physical reaction to threatening stimuli.

If a person is hiking through the woods and is surprised by an attacking bear, this direct pathway to the amygdala allows the person to begin running before he or she fully comprehends the bear. The cortex quickly presents a reality-based representation of what is occurring in the environment, but the amygdala has provided what could be a lifesaving head start.

However, the direct amygdala pathway lacks precision and may be triggered if the elements in the environment even generally approximate a previously fearful or stressful memory.[10] This pathway may become activated when we are not faced with a true survival situation and fires as a result of previous emotional learning. The direct neural wiring to the amygdala helps to explain why, in some cases, people have emotional reactions that are disproportionate to the situations at hand.

Let's return to the example of Emily. Emily is alone in her college dorm room. The campus has cleared out for that weekend. She is upset and anxious because her sextimacy partner rejected her the evening before. Finding herself alone in her room approximates events from the past, making Emily's present suffering more intense. She has a panic attack.

She finds herself deep in overwhelming emotion, with no conscious understanding of where the emotion originates. She wants to escape her room and her loneliness. One way to do this is through sextimacy. She obsessively calls her sextimacy partner, trying to reconnect with him. Although engaging in another sextimacy event is not exactly what Emily needs, she is conditioned for and intimately familiar with this emotional pattern. She unknowingly picks partners who continue this neural circuitry, whereby she feels abandoned and then she works hard to feel cared for again. Why does Emily do this? Remember, Emily did not receive any guidance for managing her emotional world—she is not skillful at consciously processing her emotional reactions (moving feelings from her amygdala to her cortex).

In this example, we see how the environment and brain circuitry interact to create an overwhelming emotional experience. Temperament, in terms of biologically predetermined tendencies, also plays an important role. Some children are more sensitive to emotion, while others are better able to tolerate and regulate their emotional experiences. Children vary in their sensitivity to emotion, but caregivers and early attachment experiences have an enormous impact on worsening or ameliorating these tendencies.

A child's understanding of her emotional world begins with how her parents react to her emotions—not only anger, frustration, and sadness, but also positive emotions. Parents may respond in ways that foster feelings of abandonment, or they may consistently respond in ways that help the child to feel cared for and safe.

Research consistently shows that parents who respond to emotions in a judgmental, punitive, or critical manner intensify their children's negative emotional experiences. This occurs because parental criticism of emotions makes a child feel bad about herself; she not only continues to feel the original negative emotion, but she loses self-esteem for having a negative emotion in the first place. Children who are judged for their emotional reactions or are left alone with their negative feelings miss the valuable opportunity to discover ways to adaptively learn how to feel better.[11]

Caregivers who approach their children's emotional world in an accepting and understanding way help children learn to treat themselves nonjudgmentally and empathically when distressed. Parents who offer warmth and acceptance for emotions, including negative ones, enable children to develop a repertoire of coping strategies. Children who receive empathy, help with problem solving, encouragement, distraction, physical comfort, or another perspective on the upsetting events are better able to manage frustration and continue with their aspirations.[12]

INCREASING YOUR FITNESS FOR DRAMA

Knowing oneself emotionally does not translate to being overly emotional. People who describe themselves as more emotionally complicated (in the sense that they have a wider range of emotional experiences and show more awareness of their own feelings) demonstrate healthier interpersonal adjustment, greater interpersonal adaptability in social situations, and greater cognitive complexity.[13] Emotional complexity is a tool that increases social awareness, and without this tool, a person will be blindsided by the actions or feelings of others. An emotionally self-aware individual is better equipped to read the expressive behavior and social cues of others. And they are better able to adjust their behavior according to specific situations.

Emotions are how the self communicates its experience of the world. If we felt nothing or were neutral, then life would hardly matter. Feelings foster an understanding of reality; they put what is important in high definition, make goals clearer, and give life genuine meaning. Emotions provide important data about preferences and core identity. Without these data, people are missing critical information about themselves. In order to manage or regulate emotions advantageously, people need to consciously reflect on what is occurring for them in the moment.

Effective emotional regulation enables people to better control impulses, tolerate frustration, delay gratification, and empathize with others. According to Daniel Goleman, author of *Emotional Intelligence*, the greater a person's ability to manage emotional experiences, the more capable he or she is to develop healthy relationships as well as to engage in successful academic and professional pursuits. As people develop a capacity for empathy and form a solid understanding for the subtleties of communication, the quality of their relationships improves.

For people to successfully manage their emotional world, it is important that they develop a belief that emotions are not fixed and uncontrollable. They actually follow a fairly predictable course. People who believe their emotions are changeable have better emotional control than people who believe emotions are uncontrollable. For example, college students who held more fixed beliefs about emotion, or believed their emotions were uncontrollable, also experienced less psychological wellbeing, increased feelings of loneliness and depression, and less social support from friends. College students who believed emotions could be changed and effectively managed adjusted better to their first year of college; they had more positive emotional experiences and experienced more social support from college friends.[14]

The remainder of this chapter is written directly to readers seeking help in changing the way they manage their emotional worlds. With these techniques, people may find that they can develop their own strategies for making themselves feel better. It is important to be flexible. There is no right way to feel, but there are approaches that help people to feel better and achieve successful long-term relationships.

HOW TO DEVELOP SELF-AWARENESS?

Healthy emotional functioning is based on attunement, or knowing what you are feeling when you are feeling it. Emotional self-awareness allows stimuli to reach the thinking area of your brain, your cortex, where conscious reflection and problem solving occur. As you become more adept at noticing your feelings, you will find that your emotions are less likely to impinge on your relational happiness.

Becoming attuned requires you to pay attention to your body and your mind. A popular and well-researched way to describe how to become more emotionally aware is through the skill of mindfulness.[15] Mindfulness is a hyper-alert awareness to the present moment and to what is occurring in the here and now. Mindfulness to emotion means training yourself to recognize subtle cues within your body. Attunement is the opposite of pushing away your emotions (or suppression), and when you do it correctly, your body remains at ease.[16]

Emotions follow a course, they come and they go, and your goal is to watch them as they travel through your nervous system. This is a process you can easily observe in young children who, without self-consciousness, display the full spectrum of their emotional worlds. As I write this, my eighteen-month-old son has a genuine passion for helicopters. When he sees one or even thinks he hears one, he becomes giddy with excitement. One day we were walking, and I heard a helicopter approach. I told my son. He squealed with delight, punched his little fist in the air, jumped up and down, and shouted at the top of his lungs, "HELICOP! HELICOP! HELICOP!" It was exhilarating to witness his joy. Within a matter of seconds, the helicopter was zooming out of sight. Pleasure drained from his face, and he began to sorrowfully wave and cry, "Bye bye, helicop, bye bye." In its simplest form, this is how our emotional processes often work. Just as we feel something and become conscious of it, it leaves us to be replaced by another emotion.

It is of utmost importance to notice the type of attention you are giving to what you are feeling. Consider whether you are self-critical, and if you are, develop open-minded labels for what you are feeling and a kind internal tone. Notice when you are using disapproving terms to describe your experience—"It is bad to feel this . . . I am weak for feeling sad . . . Why do I always feel sorry for myself?" Statements like these muddy the water and make it impossible for you to rationally assess your circumstances.

The goal is to know what you feel without losing your self-esteem in the process. Overwhelming yourself with harsh criticism prevents you from looking at specific emotions that can be identified and eventually put into perspective. As opposed to questioning what you are feeling, simply label whatever you notice—tense stomach, stress, head burning, restlessness, tears, heart pounding. Attunement requires back and forth conscious attention to what is occurring in your body, followed by labeling the feeling. The goal is to reflect—to examine your emotions without becoming engulfed by them.

Table 4.1 at the end of this chapter labels feelings, their evolutionary significance, and corresponding physical sensations. Familiarizing yourself with these labels will help you to become better skilled at knowing what you are feeling in the moment. There are three components to developing healthy emotional awareness: (1) noticing how your body is changing in reaction to emotional stimuli, (2) finding the label that best describes what you are feeling, and (3) accepting the emotion you are experiencing.[17]

Notice the Physical

There is a corresponding bodily sensation and physical urge to do something in response to nearly everything we feel. As a function of brain processes, emotions initiate adjustments in blood pressure, heart rate, muscle tension, and the digestive track. We have become so accustomed to our bodies' response to emotion that we often do not notice these sensations. By developing physical awareness, you will increase control of your reactions. It is important to tune in, from the inside out, to changes occurring in your body.

The experience of anger, for example, usually involves feeling muscles tense and an urge to lash out at someone or something. One client I worked with discovered her jaw became tight when she was angry, and as she tuned in to this, she became aware of her anger long before it got out of control and became destructive. Similarly, sadness is often accompanied by heaviness in the heart and feeling physically lethargic. Anxiety and fear may involve an increase in heart rate or tension in the gut, while pleasure often involves feeling a lack of muscle tension and a restful sensation.

Identify What You Are Feeling

The next essential component for healthy emotional attunement is your ability to choose the label that best describes what you are feeling. Many are able to do this easily, but for those who suppress their emotions, differentiating their feelings does not come without effort. Noticing sensations in your body will help you to distinguish and separate your feelings. This will let you more distinctly recognize when you are angry, sad, anxious, or happy, as well as the finer nuances between feelings. It can be helpful when stuck to ask, what is my body trying to communicate to me about how I feel in this situation? What area of my body is the most noticeable to me at this moment, and what is it signaling?

If you are jittery or keyed up, you are probably worried and anxious. If your muscles are relaxed and free of tension, you may feel pleasure. Examine how you are physically and then ask yourself if this is signaling fear, sadness, hurt, or anger. As you find the label that most aptly applies to what you are feeling, you will know it is the right one because identifying it should bring some relief.

This exercise takes practice because emotion can be a moving target. You may first notice that your heart is beating fast and you feel anxious; as soon as you label this, you may begin to notice that you feel angry toward someone, and then emerging from beneath the anger you may find hurt. Continuing to label each emotion as it comes up will help you understand much more precisely what you are experiencing, and that will enable you to cope more effectively.

The experience of anger often reflects feeling that the world is against you. People who chronically struggle with anger have both a lack of internal emotional knowledge about themselves and a lack of awareness for how their own anger plays a role in how others treat them. The quicker you recognize that it is anger you are feeling, the more likely you will be to manage the situation in an effective manner.[18]

Women, in particular, tend to turn away from anger as soon as it appears. They tell themselves that it is bad to feel anger. When anger is not consciously attended to and labeled, the risk of acting out in ways that are hurtful to others (relational aggression and bullying) increases dramatically. A person may turn the anger inward, which opens a door that often leads to depression. Anger is adaptive—evolution's way of motivating us to protect ourselves through boundary setting and self-assertion. Acknowledging anger allows a person to handle it appropriately, with his or her best interest in mind.

The typical, prominent emotion experienced with sextimacy events is sadness due to the loss of the expected personal connection. When the person involved is unaware that she is sad because of this loss, she may begin to react inappropriately. She may decide to pursue plastic surgery, become obsessively critical of her own weight, and relentlessly attack herself for lacking the social skills required to sustain male attention.

If you are feeling sad due to the loss of a relationship or sextimacy partner, it is important to label it as such. Without an accurate label, you may find that instead of identifying the loss as the problem, you come to see yourself as the problem. Once you allow yourself to feel the loss and sadness for what it is, although quite painful, you will be less likely to forge relationships with people who are unable to give you what you need.

A client who learned to recognize that she felt loss put it to me this way: "When out of nowhere he stopped talking to me I felt wounded, as if he had broken my leg and now I can't walk and he doesn't care in the least. But despite all of that I miss him . . . then I think about how hard it would be to be myself with someone who could treat me so horribly and I know that we would never be a good match." If you teach yourself to become conscious of what you are really feeling, it will help you pick a new kind of partner in the future.

Accept What You Are Feeling

Once you have a label that aptly describes your physical experience, accept that feeling. You are not trying to replay the facts of the situation, to justify or even to talk yourself out of what you are feeling. You have the feeling, and you have labeled it. It is real. Denying it would mean you are unable to know yourself on an authentic level. Even if you judge yourself harshly and push the feelings away, they will probably come out indirectly. When you indirectly express feelings that you do not understand, you may suddenly and dramatically seem to be acting inappropriately to others in your life.

Accepting your emotions is not a time to try to have empathy for the other person in the situation. Just stick with what *you* are feeling. Tell yourself that it is perfectly okay to experience whatever you are feeling. Alternatively, if you say to yourself, "I don't want this, I shouldn't feel this," or "He had a busy week, I should be more sensitive to his needs," then you are invalidating yourself.

For example, if you felt a hunger pain, would you tell yourself, "I am not hungry, I have no reason to feel hungry, I must be a pig"? I hope not. Emotions work in the same way; it is important to believe what your body and mind are telling you and to remind yourself that your experience of your life is valid. If you say, "Of course I am sad, I miss my boyfriend, and I like spending time with him," you are validating yourself. If you are angry, validate this; you can love someone and simultaneously be angry with him. Acknowledging anger in your own mind will not destroy a relationship.

The emotional workings of the brain are largely unconscious and automatic; we only know our emotions as a reality when we become conscious of a brain process that is already occurring. By attending to your physical sensations and labeling your emotions, you are moving emotional data from the amygdala to the brain's neocortex, which allows for more conscious reflection and problem solving about the emotional event. Once you are aware of what you are feeling, you can begin to look at your options for managing the feeling.

EMOTIONAL BALANCE

The goal is emotional balance. Emotional balance is a blending of *thinking* and *feeling*. It means you are neither flooded by emotion nor by rational thought. Take for example the death of a loved one—if you only *think* about this event, you might find yourself rationalizing the loss, such as, "The person was old, he or she led a good life," or "Now they are free of pain." If you continue to only *think* about the death, you will not grieve or feel sadness, which often results in feeling a lack of meaning and a sense of detachment from life. On the other hand, if all you do is *feel*, you may find that you become overwhelmed by your emotions or even depressed as a result. If you allow yourself to go in and out of both thinking and feeling, you may find you achieve a sense of acceptance and new meaning in life due to the event.

Merging emotion with intellect allows for new insights to develop, greater intimacy within yourself, and greater intimacy with others. We see this in how animals compete, as LeDoux points out: "While many animals get through life mostly on emotional automatic pilot, those animals that can readily switch from automatic pilot to willful control have a tremendous extra advantage. This advantage depends on the wedding of emotional and cognitive functions."[19]

Though at first glance blending thinking and feeling may seem an easy task, our neuroanatomy does not readily integrate the emotional and the cognitive. People often report *knowing* something to be true ("This guy is no good for me") and yet *feeling* quite differently ("but I can't stop myself from wanting to be with him"). One reason for this may be that there is a clear anatomical divide in the brain between emotion and rational thinking. Because the emotional centers of the brain evolved long before the thinking areas, the brain is wired in such a way that emotions can flood our thinking. We can certainly influence this divide, but in order to do so, we must consciously reflect on our emotions; without this conscious attention, emotions will dominate every aspect of our behavior.

As described earlier in this chapter, fearful emotional data can bypass the neocortex. The amygdala has a wide network of connections that are primitive and potent. When activated by an intense and fearful emotional trigger, the emotional pathways will permeate the thinking areas of the brain so that you cannot think rationally. As Goleman explains:

> One drawback of such neural alarms is that the urgent message the amygdala sends is sometimes, if not often, out of date—especially in the fluid social world we humans inhabit. As the repository for emotional memory, the amygdala scans experience, comparing what is happening now with what happened in the past. Its method of comparison is associative: when one key element of a present situation is similar to the past, it can call it a "match"—which is why this circuit is sloppy: it acts before there is full confirmation. It frantically commands that we react to the present in ways that were imprinted long ago, with thoughts, emotions, reactions learned in response to events perhaps only dimly similar, but close enough to alarm the amygdala.[20]

The direct amygdala pathway makes black and white judgments about experiences: healthy or harmful, good or bad, fair or unfair, safe or unsafe. Important nuance is missed when the facts of a situation do not match the intense emotion experienced. In this case and many others, we need the help of our neocortex to grasp this nuance and bring it to our conscious awareness.

Imagine standing in the check-out line at a grocery store while the impatient shopper behind you repeatedly bumps you with his cart. If you allow your amygdala to dominate, you may feel rage. You might reflexively push back and make a threat without considering the consequences of escalating a confrontation with such a dubious character.

The prefrontal cortex, mercifully, has the ability to soothe the amygdala and regulate an emotional reaction.[21] The frontal cortex acts as a conductor of many instruments and works to analyze, problem solve, and consider various perspectives. Because the neural wiring is more intricate, the frontal lobe takes longer to respond than the amygdala. Once it takes over, the frontal lobe is your friend and will help you to feel better. The final section of this chapter provides empirically based and effective methods for accessing your frontal lobe and achieving emotional balance.[22]

WHAT DO YOU WANT TO DO?

Imagine you have a superb first date with a new romantic interest, and you feel entirely absorbed by his personality and charm. You may even fleetingly feel as if you are falling in love with this person. Your cortex should be telling you that this is a *feeling* not based on multiple experiences over time with the individual. If you do not access your cortex, you may find yourself blissfully telling the person, "I love you!"

As much as possible, it is important not to act without first reflecting. Taking a day or even a few moments to reflect before acting gives your cortex time to catch up, so you may more thoughtfully respond to the developing circumstances.

Our ways of responding to emotion (particularly fear) can be extremely primitive at times, and if we allow ourselves to always go with the feeling, we sharply limit ourselves. For example, if you have a fear of anything (flying, elevators, or heights), the psychotherapy treatment of choice is typically some variant of what is termed exposure therapy. The premise of this treatment approach is to help you become comfortable doing the thing you fear most, simply by getting you to do it over and over again. Exposure therapy is based on the idea that new learning occurs when habitual ways of responding are blocked. By doing the opposite of what you feel like doing in the moment, you will alter your perception of the emotional event. When you no longer engage in the same old behavior, you give your frontal lobe a chance to chime in and help you cope more effectively. This sets the stage for you to develop a new mental habit that, over time, will become automatic.

Negative feelings can often be relieved through forcing yourself to do exactly what you least feel like doing.[23] When you are depressed, you may have the desire to be alone, to do nothing, to be a couch potato. Instead, do that which feels the hardest to do in that moment—go against what your feeling is telling you to do. If lonely, force yourself to be around others, go to a crowded event, interact. If you are afraid to be yourself in relationships, force yourself to talk about yourself again and again in social situations.

WHAT ARE YOU THINKING?

This aspect of emotional regulation has to do with the story you are telling yourself about the situation that is causing your emotional reaction. Research literature consistently finds that reappraisal works wonders to make people feel better. Reappraisal is changing the way you think about what is distressing you. This may occur by finding enhanced meaning, a clearer purpose, or a more certain direction from what is upsetting. Reappraisal also works through looking at the facts in a different way or by reminding yourself of your longer-term goals.

Reappraisal is the gold standard when it comes to ways to make yourself feel better. Oliver John and James Gross, leading researchers in the area of emotion regulation, found that relying on reappraisal as a way to regulate emotion is related to feeling better overall and to better interpersonal functioning.[24] Even when people are seriously physically ill, finding meaning helps them to feel better. For example, breast cancer patients who find positive meaning (believe the illness changed what they value in life or helped them to develop a more positive outlook) fare better in terms of psychologically adjusting to both the disease and also to the treatment.[25]

When you realize you are upset by something, notice what that little voice inside your head is saying about the event. Chances are it is saying something that is aggravating the wound, reminding you of why you are hurt, or replaying similarly troubling events from your past. As discussed earlier, emotion easily floods the thinking areas of the brain, distorting the facts of a situation so that you are not thinking rationally about what has occurred. Notice when your thoughts are intensifying the negative emotion you feel.

For reappraisal to work, you cannot just make up a story or rationalize what occurred. Reappraisal is neither a romanticized version nor a worst-case interpretation of the emotional event, but one that is based on the facts, both good and bad. Imagine you have been casually seeing someone with whom you have become enamored, and he tells you that he is not ready for a real relationship. Perhaps you find yourself swimming in disappointment and hurt. If you continue to tell yourself the worst-case scenario, your feelings will intensify, and you may find yourself engaging in self-defeating behavior, such as starting another sextimacy relationship or calling the guy and criticizing him. If you romanticize the story to make yourself feel better and tell yourself that if you just hang in there long enough, your specialness will surely win him over, then you are not dealing with reality, and you are setting yourself up for additional hurt. A realistic reappraisal of this situation might be something like, "Better to find out now before I became more serious with him," or "People vary in terms of when they are ready for a relationship, and this is not always something personal about me." You may even remind yourself that to have a successful partnership, you need someone who is mature enough to say he wants a relationship.

If you are struggling to find an objective way to mentally reframe an upsetting emotional event, imagine a friend came to you with the exact same predicament. In working to give her an objective appraisal of the situation, what would you tell her? In addition, as you talk to yourself, use a soothing, gentle, calm voice, just as a good caretaker or caring friend would. Remember to treat yourself compassionately as you notice what is real or what might be distorted in the story you are telling yourself.

Reappraisal works best if it occurs as close as possible to when you first experience the upsetting emotion. It is harder to rethink something if your blood is boiling in upset or if you are firmly in denial. In other words, try to reappraise before emotions become too overwhelming or are avoided altogether. As soon as you get a hint (tense muscles, sickness in the pit of your stomach, increased heart rate) that something is bothering you, stop and ask what you are saying to yourself about the event. Then find a new way to think about the event, a new story that is compassionately realistic.

LONG-TERM CONTENTMENT

Clinicians have long observed a relationship between feeling emotionally depleted and engaging in self-defeating or even self-destructive behaviors. In an effort to understand this relationship, social science researchers conducted a series of laboratory experiments where research participants were offered a choice between two lotteries: Lottery A promised a 70 percent chance of winning a $2 prize; lottery B offered a 4 percent chance of winning a $25 prize. Lottery A was a low-risk way to win $2 while lottery B was plainly the riskier option.

Those participants who experienced a negative emotional state in the laboratory were more likely to choose the riskier lottery than those participants in a neutral mood state. Picking the riskier option meant these participants essentially ignored relevant data that they were unlikely to actually win such a lottery. Even though they were substantially more likely to encounter a bad outcome, they were willing to risk this for the tiny chance that they might gain a higher payoff.[26]

This study and others like it suggest that an unhappy mood makes a person more susceptible to risky choices. Researchers theorize that people in a negative mood already feel so poorly and depleted that another risk is irrelevant to them. They tend to focus on the possibility, no matter how small, that a major mood boost might occur—an appealing gamble when experiencing a depleted self.

People who are emotionally distressed are more vulnerable to risky behaviors that offer a small chance of a high reward. Occasionally the high-payoff/high-risk option works, as is the case with a briefly fulfilling sextimacy encounter that offers a temporary mood boost. Over the long run, risky wagers do not deliver. Similarly, over the long term, a sextimacy encounter leaves women feeling more emotionally depleted than before the event occurred. If you are emotionally depleted, you are more at risk for self-defeating decisions, including sextimacy.

It is important when you are in a negative mood to remind yourself of your longer-term self-esteem and relationship goals. In the study discussed above, researchers went back and told those participants in a negative mood state to "Think carefully about their decision" before making it. This reminder, to reflect before making a choice, all but eliminated the trend for participants in negative mood states to make riskier choices. When you experience a depleted mood, remind yourself that you must consciously think through your choices; careful consideration decreases the tendency to make risky decisions that are not in your long-term best interest.

STOMACH IT

No matter what you tell yourself or what you do, you may find that you continue to feel emotional pain. The truth is there are moments when you just have to feel bad for a period of time and accept that life is not always rosy. You would not expect to go through life and never feel physically sick. Negative feelings, including anger, a desire to be mean, jealousy, worry, and sadness, are all normal parts of the human condition and give you key information about yourself and your relationships. Allow yourself to just sit with whatever you are feeling. Label it. Remind yourself that it will pass.

As hard as it is to experience pain or hurt, once you successfully bear it, you may find the feeling propels you toward a clear goal or direction. At times, feeling your pain will enable you to chart a course that is ultimately more fulfilling. When Emily allowed herself to fully experience the hurt she felt with inconsistent and unpredictable sextimacy partners, she eventually reconnected with her childhood pain of feeling she was an emotional burden to her parents. Emily forged healthier connections with men through developing awareness for these past relationship dynamics and recognizing how her childhood hurt influences her current relationships.

If you continually tell yourself that everything is fine, even when you are drowning inside, you never give yourself the opportunity to clean things up and make a positive change. When you are out of touch with what troubles you, it becomes impossible to build healthy relationships.

SHINE THE SPOTLIGHT

Consider your attention span to be a spotlight. You are only able to see where you shine the light. To get a full picture, you must move the spotlight around. If you fail to move the light, you will miss important information about what you are feeling and what others feel about you. It is missing that information that leaves you vulnerable and shocked when others express negative feelings toward you.

Notice where you aim your spotlight and keep it in balance. Attend to what you are feeling in the moment as well as the bigger picture of your life. Consider if you become bogged down in emotion and if you do, distract yourself, leave the situation mentally for a period of time and then revisit it with a new perspective. Take note if you are overly attending to trivial details in your world, such as a perceived physical flaw or whether a guy will call you back. Ruminating and overthinking trivial matters signals a need to refocus your attention on emotions you may be suppressing.

INCREASE PLEASURE

Pleasure is an elixir and has the potential to soothe even the most aggravating of emotional experiences. It would seem to be axiomatic, but in the midst of turmoil, it serves to remind that the more you increase your positive experiences and allow yourself to feel pleasure, the easier it will be to manage your more difficult feelings. Researchers have long observed an association between positive experiences and psychological resiliency. Those who have enjoyable experiences to look forward to are less prone to depression and tend to more easily rebound from negative emotions.[27]

A higher ratio of pleasurable experiences in your life not only leads to more positive mood states, but also contributes to better problem solving and effective emotional coping. When researchers induce a positive mood state in research participants, participants demonstrate a better attention span, increased working memory, and a greater awareness of the information presented.[28] Increased working memory serves as a buffer against less effective coping strategies, particularly rumination, because it makes it possible to consider a wider range of coping tactics. If something bothers you and you distract yourself with something pleasurable, you may find that when you return to what was bothersome, you have a clearer perspective.

CONDUCT A COST-BENEFIT ANALYSIS

Another important tool that helps people to feel better is problem solving. Problem solving is a deliberate consideration of your options for managing the difficult emotion experienced. Instead of telling yourself, "I feel horrible and will feel this forever," problem solving is a way to view the specific situation at hand and choose actions that will bring relief.

To effectively problem solve, write down possible ways to manage the feelings you are experiencing, and then imagine how the scenarios might play out and how you would feel if each actually occurred. Conduct a cost-benefit analysis by thinking through the consequences and benefits to you of each method for handling your emotional reaction.

For example, if you feel hurt in a relationship, you may be conflicted about whether to tell the person how he hurt you, to tell someone who is uninvolved in the situation, or to keep the hurt feelings to yourself. Consider what the costs and benefits will be to you for each of these possibilities: (1) Telling the person who hurt you may encourage him to be more sensitive next time and even increase your intimacy. On the other hand, it may intensify the conflict. (2) Telling someone who is uninvolved may provide an immediate emotional release but is not going to directly address the underlying problem. (3) Stomaching the emotion and holding your feelings inside may help you to maintain the relationship, but you may continue to feel distress.

Decide which cost you are most willing to accept and which option brings you closer to your long-term intent. If your goal is to find a partner with whom you can be emotionally honest, then it will behoove you to speak directly to him if he hurts you. If you have too many hurt feelings in relationships, and your goal is to not overburden your partners, then speaking to someone uninvolved may be effective.

Problem solving is best begun immediately, but at times it can be difficult because the emotion experienced is so intense. In these cases, it can be helpful to let some time pass. Attenuate your negative emotion by using one of the other strategies described: reappraisal, increase pleasure, or shine the spotlight. Then mentally revisit the problematic situation. Allowing yourself to feel an emotion after the fact is similar to receiving an inoculation. By offering your brain a less virulent strain of the original negative emotion, you have an opportunity to thoughtfully consider the events and anticipate how you will manage the situation more effectively next time (there is always a next time). Play the event forward, imagining how you would prefer it to go in the future. What do you wish you had done differently? How do you think about the situation now compared to when it first occurred?

To keep problem solving from devolving into rumination, ask yourself what you can actively do to manage the problem and put a time limit on the exercise. Once your allotted time is up, let it rest. Distract or throw yourself into something else; otherwise, you may be vulnerable to unproductive rumination.

EXPRESS YOUR FEELINGS

Whether it is the person who upset you or a kind and supportive friend, spouse, or caregiver, often there is truly nothing more relieving than simply telling another human being about your distress. Many research studies demonstrate the benefits of talking and letting your feelings out with another person. Psychotherapy is designed on the basic premise that speaking with someone about what hurts helps people to feel more in control and less afraid of what they feel. The act of talking, labeling, and expressing moves emotional information to your cortex and will help you feel better.

It is important to choose the right person with whom to discuss your feelings. If you choose someone who is a conflictual person within the specific situation, then it will likely add to the negative emotion you are experiencing. Emotional relief can even come by talking with others with whom you have very little intimacy or do not know well. In one study, when research participants felt intense feelings of rejection and then talked online with someone they did not even know, they actually felt more accepted, and their self-esteem improved.[29]

The feelings of rejection or abandonment, two key emotions that propel the sextimacy cycle, are often accompanied by a physical urge to be alone where self-banishment and self-abuse ensue. Interacting and talking with others provides a new experience that counters feeling rejected.

CONCLUSION

Of course, expressing your feelings is not always the effective course of action and is entirely dependent on the social demands of the situation. If you are in a work meeting and express to your boss, "I hate you," she may fire you. However, in the context of relationships and sextimacy, communicating your feelings is vital for picking the right partner and for effectively managing the relationship. In the next chapter, we will closely assess when you need to communicate and how to do it effectively.

SELF-ASSESSMENT: DO YOU AVOID EMOTION?

Take this self-assessment to find out if you allow yourself to feel your emotions or if you avoid emotion. The more yeses you have, the more likely you may be to being blindsided by life events like breakups, divorce, job loss, and general breaches in relationships that are upsetting and surprising to you. If you dismiss and minimize your in-the-moment emotional experiences, you lose touch with who you are as a person and become out of touch with the motives and feelings of others. The more items you endorse, the more you need to increase your emotional self-awareness.

1. If you cry, you are weak.
2. Women who talk about their feelings are drama queens.
3. Even if I was irate with someone, I would make sure to put on a smile.
4. People need to buck up and stop feeling sorry for themselves.
5. When people talk about their feelings, they are just making things worse.
6. Feelings should not be taken seriously.
7. I am often surprised by my emotions.

8. Whenever I cry, I know I am being stupid.
9. Emotions are black and white; it is women who make them complicated.
10. As long as I stay busy, feelings don't really bother me.
11. When men cry, I want to puke.
12. If I feel bad, I tell myself to get over it and be a big girl.
13. When my friends are upset, I criticize them.
14. When upset, I just move on to the next thing and shrug it off.
15. I feel better if I just tell myself to not think about what is upsetting me.
16. I regularly tell myself that if I think positively, I will be happy.
17. People who pay attention to how they feel about things are overly dramatic and not to be taken seriously.
18. When my friends are upset, I remind them of how lucky they are and all that they have in their lives.
19. I prefer to be around men; women are too emotional.
20. I pride myself on always being the logical one in the group.

It may seem surprising, but some people have difficulty knowing what they are feeling in the moment. If you experience this problem, use table 4.1 as an aid in labeling what it is you are *really* feeling.

Table 4.1.

FEELINGS

Emotions	Physical/Bodily Sensations	Labels to Describe Your Experience	Action Urges	Evolutionary Significance
Love	Body feels calm, muscles relaxed, sense of internal peace, wellbeing	Sense of comfort, safety, comfort with another, passion, sexual longing	Desire to be with the person, to bond with the other, wanting to make sure the other is okay	Love binds couples, children, families, and tribes together. It is the glue that connects people.
Pleasure	Accompanied by the brain releasing "feel-good hormones," so you may feel increased energy, lack of physical pain; body is excited	Delight, joy, vivaciousness, contentment, mastery, lost in the moment, not thinking about the future or the past	Urge to smile, laugh, talk more with others, and reveal more about yourself	Pleasure is a tonic for negative emotions and motivates us to do certain things so that we may experience more pleasure.
Anger	Body feels tense, jaw clinches, muscles tighten, increased body temperature, pressure behind the eyes	Feeling unfairly treated or disrespected by others or the world as a whole, outrage, rage, feeling the self is not valued	Urge to lash out, or harm another; urge to yell at someone, throw something	Anger cues the body to self-protect through physical force, self-assertion, or boundary setting.

Sadness	Body wants to remain still; feeling lethargic, a lack of energy, may be hard to get your body to move	Loss, grief, hopelessness, rejection, feeling defeated or unwanted by others, feeling bad about the self	Urge to cry, sit still or in one place; lack of motivation; urge to ruminate about what you did to cause the loss	Sadness is protective in that it allows the self to sit in place while grief and problem solving can take place.
Anxiety	Brain triggers the stress hormones that cause muscle tension, restlessness, increased heartbeat, sweating, shortness of breath, stomachache	Worried, fearful, feeling threatened by something in the environment or within a relationship (fear of losing a relationship); on high alert, vigilant, survival mode	Urge to be vigilant, replay events in one's mind, predict future events; desire to take control of the threat; urge to flee or to busy the self	Anxiety triggers adrenaline so that the body goes into high alert. You become primed for action and protection.
Guilt	Body feels sick, stomach hurts, muscles hurt; feels as if you can't be physically at ease	Feeling like a "bad" person, feeling destructive, feeling you should be punished	Urge to make amends, to be a "better" person; urge to berate the self	Guilt keeps people in accordance with societal laws designed for protecting people.
Shame	Burning sensation on the face, cheeks flush, stomach sinking	Embarrassment, humiliation, fearing exposure as a fraud, that a flaw will be revealed to another or to the public	Urge to flee or leave the situation, to become invisible, to hide the self from others	Shame signifies social status in a group and keeps people in accordance with group expectations.

Source: R. Plutchik (2002). *Emotions and Life: Perspectives from Psychology, Biology, and Evolution*. Washington, DC: American Psychological Association.

5

CHATTERBOX

Building Direct Communication

The label *fake* is a common put-down used by women to describe another woman who communicates a disingenuous air of niceness. For most women, there is a fine line between what they privately know to be true and what they choose to openly communicate to others. Girls are socialized to become acutely concerned with what to say and when to say it and to protect the feelings of others. Because most women function within these cultural constraints, they easily imagine that other women are hiding their private or less socially desirable thoughts and feelings.

Girls and women are stymied by the cultural expectation that they are to be perpetually pleasing to others. The degree to which women choose not to express their true selves is profound and may impact every aspect of a woman's identity. One recent study reports that 80 percent of women fake orgasms, and most of these women report doing so in order to increase their partner's self-esteem.[1] This is striking evidence of how much women will fake in order to ensure that others are content.

So culture places girls and women in a dilemma in terms of language and communication. They are fully qualified to speak, but unless they carefully edit what they say, they may be judged harshly. *Chatterbox*, *drama queen*, *princess*, *diva*, *manipulator*, and other labels constrain girls from becoming too much themselves or too unabashedly expressive.

There is a lasting impact on a little girl's understanding of herself if, when communicating, she is told that she is "articulate," as opposed to being told that she "talks too much." When judgmental and stereotypical language is applied to a girl, it narrows her understanding of herself. If when a girl becomes emotional she is labeled a *drama queen*, then she feels this judgment and in some respect curtails her effort to communicate frankly. If a girl who can speak her mind clearly and with confidence is labeled a *chatterbox*, her confidence will be undermined.

Language informs the way we think and understand the world, as well as how we understand ourselves. Language may provide individuals with wide possibility or reduce them to halting stereotypes. When women allow themselves to speak their minds, they are able to change not only a single relationship but also their world.

THE EVOLUTION OF LANGUAGE

Primates have varied and creative ways of communicating. They gesture, pantomime, grunt, and combine various sounds. Researchers observed chimpanzees in the Ugandan Budongo Forest and discovered that chimps alter the pitch of their screams according to whether they are a victim or an aggressor within a conflict. As Christine Kenneally describes in her compelling book *The First Word*, "The researcher witnessed one exchange in which a young male was harassing a female chimp that was giving loud victim screams in response. At one point . . . the female had clearly had enough and began instead to make aggressor screams back at the young male. She was then joined by another female in retaliating against the male. The second female appeared from out of sight, so she must have used the information in the first female's scream to make her decision."[2] The recordings of the chimps' screams demonstrated it was possible to discern, solely from the screams, whether the chimps were in high-risk situations or low-risk situations. Researchers found that in high-risk situations, the chimps' screams were long and high-pitched, while in less risky situations, the screams tended to be shorter and lower in pitch. Help bounds forward for the chimps in need as a result of a change in the pitch of their screams.

Human language has evolved to become the elegant and sophisticated machine it is today. Long gone are the days of grunting and pantomiming; human language allows us to communicate fine-grain detail, bringing to life the most complicated of inner experiences or creative ideas. Without a complex language, the advancement of human culture through creative innovation is unimaginable. Language is essential for our survival, reproduction, and general advancement of the species. As Kenneally observes, "If some global disaster killed all humans, there would be no language left. If language suddenly became inaccessible to us, perhaps we would all die, too."[3]

Language is the only medium through which we become less alone with our private experiences of the world. The simple act of talking about our experiences, whether it is about constructing a railroad or managing conflict in a relationship, changes the way we think and feel about these same experiences. Language offers a release for painful emotions, protecting against the unchallenged havoc of anxiety and depression. If people are unable or unwilling to use their voices effectively, then they are at a deficit in terms of being able to understand themselves as well as the world around them. While the power of language is palpable and the human capacity for artful communication is limitless, there are social and cultural blocks to women fully utilizing this valuable resource.

LOST VOICE

By adolescence, many girls no longer use their voice to communicate what is real for them but curtail what they say only to that which maintains their relationships. As Lyn Mikel Brown, author of *Girlfighting*, observes, "First we tell girls to attend to relationships, and then we expect them to take their own strong feelings out of relationships to protect the feelings of others or to maintain a cover story of girls as nice and 'friends to everybody.'"[4] The reasons for this loss of voice relate to the tendency to socialize girls toward niceness, politeness, and compulsive attentiveness to the feelings of others. Girls enter their relationships with a lack of preparedness for effectively managing normative conflict and feel they have only two options—either play nice or lose a friend/

romantic partner. Without any skills for managing conflict, many girls and women believe they are flawed if they do not live up to the idealistic expectation of continual relationship bliss. Faced with the possibility of feeling inherently flawed and unlovable, girls choose to mask what they think and feel to ensure their relationships will continue.

In an effort to guarantee that they do not directly voice their upset to others, women may minimize their distress through invalidating themselves. When faced with conflict or negative emotion, some women and girls simply tell themselves that what they are thinking or feeling is not real. They ardently work to convince themselves that the negative emotion they are feeling is unjustified, unwarranted, or illogical given the facts of the situation. Examples of this include, "I do not know why I am upset; this is really no big deal . . . I am only upset because I have my period . . . I am emotional because I am really hormonal right now . . . I just need to stop being so dramatic . . . I am acting like such a girl; there really is nothing to be upset about."

Another way women avoid voicing their negative feelings to others is by becoming absorbed in the story of their partner and consumed by feelings of empathy. One client, Cindy, often felt disappointed and resentful when her sextimacy partner would suddenly drop out of contact for weeks at a time. When he would resurface, she did not communicate her justified feelings of upset to him but instead listened empathically as he described his work stress.

Research suggests that while men tend to limit what they express to remain in control and have power in their relationships, women are less expressive of certain emotions so as not to damage their relationships.[5] As a result, many women choose to maintain relationships that are unhealthy or do not match their long-term goals. This is where sextimacy thrives, as the woman never directly voices her negative feelings, and the man is never held accountable. An example of this is the dynamic in which the woman in a relationship builds her self-worth around the project of becoming closer to a withdrawn and emotionally unavailable man. This project allows the male figure in the relationship to develop closeness with his partner on his terms but leaves the woman feeling disappointed and unfulfilled as her needs for emotional intimacy go unmet.

Rather than focusing on the healthiness of the relationship itself, many women who are unhappy with this type of arrangement turn their unhappiness on themselves through painful self-criticism. When relationships sour, women become self-critical because deep down they believe good girls have relationships that are filled only with sugar and spice, and anything less is their fault. Girls and women who lose their voice for communicating the full range of their feelings in relationships are vulnerable to prolonging dysfunctional relationships.

The socialization many women receive trains them to, above all else, maintain their relationships, and so women learn to suppress, repress, or deny feelings of anger when mistreated by another. When they legitimately do feel anger, some women learn to voice that they are feeling stressed, sad, or tired because these feelings are less likely to cause direct conflict.

This is seen in the case of Rachel, a forty-four-year-old client who was in the process of recognizing that her husband of fifteen years was having an affair, which had extended over the previous five years. Rachel was a working mother of two children; she put her husband through medical school and easily accepted his trips away from the family for "work" events. Although she resented him for his frequent absences, she pushed away feeling angry and convinced herself she was stressed by work and child demands. When she was forced to confront her husband, she felt her life's work collapsing around her, and anger occasionally made an appearance.

During our sessions, Rachel would occasionally clench her fist as she described feeling stressed by friends who discussed her husband's affair. When I asked her, "Are you angry at your husband for what has happened? Does it feel fair to you?," she would, without hesitation, look at me with surprise and respond, "Angry? No, not angry, more just hurt . . . " And so it went for six months until one day, while dutifully packing up her husband's belongings, she saw a photo of her children laughing and playing in their pool. She knew her children would never have that kind of security and ease in their lives again, and for the first time she felt anger. She felt enraged that her husband was willing to cavalierly throw away that for which she worked so hard and to flatly deny her needs and those of her children. The anger was overwhelming, but it led

Rachel to a new awareness about herself and what she would no longer tolerate from others. By allowing herself to communicate this anger to her husband, Rachel began to develop a backbone, and her husband was forced to hear her voice.

While men tend to express their anger directly to the person who evokes their displeasure, women tend to communicate their anger to others who are uninvolved in the situation.[6] Because they are afraid anger will rupture their relationships, girls and women are more likely to smile and keep the positive feelings flowing than to directly express negative feelings to the offender. Nonetheless, like all emotions, anger needs a release, and when complicated feelings are not communicated, they emerge in other ways. For many girls and women, this takes the form of relational aggression or bullying. Relational aggression is favored because, on the surface, it appears as though there has been no purposeful wrongdoing at all.[7] Gossip, manipulation, and passive aggressive behaviors are ways some women communicate anger that they cannot allow themselves to directly voice.

One of the consequences of socializing girls toward "niceness" in their relationships is that they are left ill-prepared when it comes to interpersonal friction. In Rachel Simmons's interviews for *Odd Girl Out*, adolescent girls stated again and again that they do not directly discuss their negative feelings with other girls (and presumably we can extend this to sextimacy partners where needs for connection are firmly at play) out of fear that it will hurt someone's feelings or cause a relationship to end. It is an interesting paradox that develops when girls and women protect their relationships by not communicating negative opinions directly. In actuality, it is indirect communication, bullying, passive aggressive behavior, and gossip that hurt women's feelings and lead to less intimacy in relationships.

In the moment, gossip works wonders for managing anger. When conflict presents itself, the woman may focus on someone else altogether, feel better about herself, and ensure her safety within the group.[8] However, relational aggression leaves little opportunity for real intimacy or authenticity with others.

For some, communicating to another person, "I am angry with you," is so threatening that they choose to label their angry feelings as hurt or stress and, as such, avoid the dreaded word—anger. When inauthentic feelings are communicated to others, self-esteem and the respect of others diminish. Choosing to keep a cool exterior through hiding one's anger and expressing fake feelings causes a striking sacrifice of self where a person loses control of his or her destiny.

Women who are able to directly voice anger in their relationships actually have increased intimacy with others and higher self-esteem. Directly communicating anger often allows for the development of healthier boundaries in relationships and helps others to know what is needed from them. In the longer term, directly voicing anger often changes the power dynamic of a relationship, enhances relationship satisfaction, and increases self-esteem. Appropriately expressing anger may cause a particular relationship to end but opens the door for a more fulfilling future partnership.

Some women also have difficulty communicating their positive feelings about themselves. They are conditioned to discuss themselves in a modest and nonassertive manner and likewise develop beliefs that it is bad to brag. Women tend to suppress feeling good about themselves to avoid giving voice to prideful feelings, thus ensuring they do not somehow make another person feel uncomfortable.[9]

Women and girls often judge or gossip when one of their own directly communicates her accomplishments or sources of pride. When I asked a bright teenage girl why she never told her friends about her academic successes, she replied, "I don't want to look like I think I am *all that*." Over time, girls and women begin to unconsciously feel it is not feminine to directly voice accomplishment or to outwardly demonstrate areas of strength. Too many girls and women let others know of their sources of pride in indirect ways, through self-deprecating remarks or compulsively adding caveats like, "I just got really lucky on this one." Modesty and self-deprecation are sociably desirable traits, but some women come to believe that their accomplishments are not of value.

WHY MUST WE COMMUNICATE?

When private thoughts are communicated, it is not surprising that relationships may change. They may change for the better by bringing increased closeness or intimacy to the relationship. Alternatively, a woman may find that a relationship she is holding on to is simply not salvageable. This last possibility is what often deters women from communicating their more assertive or negative feelings.

It can be helpful to recognize that denying to oneself that a relationship is dysfunctional has far greater consequences than confronting it head on. As one study found, wives with poorer communication abilities were more likely to be psychologically abused by their husbands.[10] When people do not speak of their anger or assert themselves emotionally, they become vulnerable to maintaining relationships that are one sided.

One other important note is that research shows people are attracted to those who are on par with their own communication abilities. This means that if you have difficulty communicating, you may be attracted to others who also have impaired communication skills and less attracted to those who have the ability to communicate better than you do.[11] Many couples are stuck in a recurrent dysfunctional communication pattern simply because neither partner communicates very well.

If you have difficulty directly communicating your internal thoughts, you are likely vulnerable to developing relationships with poor communicators. Poor communicators often rely on expressing their feelings in a physical or sexual manner, which makes it hard for a relationship to deepen. It is important to work on your communication abilities before picking your Prince Charming so that you may be attracted to a more effective communicator.

Speaking is not entirely an innate ability. Children do not learn language if they do not hear it spoken and are not around others whom they may verbally imitate. And refining effective language skills is an ongoing process. Thought and even practice can dramatically improve communication. The remainder of this chapter is written directly to readers who want to develop more effective communication patterns within their relationships.

IMPAIRED COMMUNICATION AS A TURN-ON

When direct communication is poor between romantic partners, as is often the case with sextimacy, each is left to feel insecure about the status of the relationship. Although feelings of insecurity and fear are signs that the relationship is unhealthy, perversely, these feelings often compel couples to feel more invested in and enthralled by one another—at least temporarily.

For example, in one well-known study researchers asked male participants to cross a stable or unstable bridge where a male or female research assistant met them. Once across the bridge, they were provided with the research assistant's phone number and asked to write a brief story. Male participants who crossed the unstable bridge were more likely than those who crossed the stable bridge to both include greater sexual imagery in their stories and to call the female research assistant at her home. Researchers concluded that the fear and arousal the men felt while crossing the unstable bridge resulted in a feeling of attraction for the female assistants.[12]

This study and others like it suggest that certain negative emotions, including fear, can cause a person to feel greater attraction to a partner. Similar to the feelings a roller coaster evokes, heated arguments and highly conflictual communication patterns between partners create simultaneous feelings of fear and arousal. Although at first many experience this roller coaster as attraction and closeness, over time dysfunctional communication is a libido killer.

In another example, some women are attracted to men who communicate an air of aloofness and arrogance, even though in the long run these traits are antithetical to a mutually fulfilling relationship. In one study, a group of male actors was asked to either comport themselves in a dominant manner (sitting in a very casual way while speaking loudly and exhibiting little interest in the women present) or nondominant manner (sitting up straight and speaking quietly).[13] Women reported being more attracted to those men who behaved in a dominant manner. Strong traits of control and power, although perhaps sexy to some, are not associated with being communicative, kind, or empathetic.[14]

MUTUAL COMMUNICATION

Typically women feel the psychological responsibility for making sure their relationships are running smoothly and progressing. When in a romantic relationship, women are more likely to initiate difficult conversations, express vulnerable emotions, and ask questions about the status or future of the relationship. While women work hard to keep their relationships intact, they all too often settle for men who, in terms of communication, do not reciprocate. Some ignore it when the man indirectly communicates that he is intimacy avoidant. This occurs because women suffer a loss of self-esteem when their relationships do not work out. One result is sextimacy, where the woman continually wishes for increased closeness while the man works to keep closeness away.

Healthy relationship development with intimacy is dependent on mutually communicating feelings regarding the relationship. Directly communicating where you are is important, and equally important is hearing and accepting where the other person is in the relationship. If you tell a partner you are really falling for him and he looks away, makes a sarcastic comment, or begins joking or roughhousing with you, he is communicating that he is either unable or unwilling to reciprocate your level of intimacy. Similarly, if you have been with someone for more than a few months and he cannot directly state that he wants to be with you or really likes you, then the relationship is not progressing.

Genuine emotional closeness cannot be maintained if only one person is doing the work of expressing emotion and intimacy within the relationship. It is critical that intimate interactions be reciprocated. In order for a relationship to be fulfilling, the man must be able to both express his more private thoughts about the relationship and respond favorably to your expressions of closeness. Research suggests that when men truly fall in love, they are verbally communicative about how they feel in the relationship. As a matter of fact, when a relationship is the right match for men, they are typically the first to say, "I love you," and they *verbally* communicate their general affection.[15]

SELF-DISCLOSURE

Self-disclosure is the most far-reaching way people communicate about who they are. When a relationship is just beginning, it may feel comfortable only to disclose surface aspects of your personality, such as where you are from, your job, or your social acquaintances. With time and if the relationship is healthy, you should feel at ease disclosing information about your family history, childhood experiences, and eventually even imperfect personality traits. Intimate and fulfilled couples tend to listen attentively to one another's self-disclosures. Close couples feel that few topics are off limits, and an open dialogue permeates their relationship. There are two primary relationship dynamics that suggest a relationship has no shot of ever evolving to mutual intimacy.

The first dynamic is termed "Game Playing Love," whereby one member of the couple approaches the relationship in a more fun and casual manner.[16] The game player looks to love for immediate gratification but not for lasting commitment. Game players keep their romantic partners at a distance so that they may continue to date around and not feel committed. Typically, because women generally have a stronger drive for intimacy and authentic relationships, the game player in the relationship is the man. Game-playing men consistently put their self-interests before their relationships. They keep most conversation with their partners on a superficial level. Rather than self-disclose, game players exclusively engage their romantic partners through activities—playing racquetball every night; constantly going to movies, concerts, and sporting events; or meeting up at local bars. Game players have difficulty verbally communicating about themselves in an authentic manner and so are hesitant, if not altogether unwilling, to reveal much detail about their inner lives. By keeping partners at a distance and by not disclosing much about himself, the game player protects himself against the criticism that might come with being known, flaws and all.

Women who are dealing with game players typically respond by working even harder to foster intimacy. This is a self-defeating strategy: The harder the woman works, the further away the game player moves because intimacy for him is Kryptonite. Women who are partnered with game players often make excuses for the superficiality in the relationship—"He had a difficult childhood . . . I know he cares about me because I can just feel it . . . He shows his care for me in different ways . . . I should trust him and feel more secure." They may hold onto one shining example where the game player was romantic and emotionally demonstrative. These are rationalizations for feeling unknown and unwanted by one's partner. Game-playing love ultimately leaves the woman with a lack of self-respect for tolerating a relationship that does not fulfill her.

The second communication dynamic that is not conducive to verbal intimacy over the long term is the "Stranger on the Plane" phenomenon.[17] Perhaps you have sat next to someone while traveling who has shown you pictures of his grandchildren, described his difficulty finding a job, and talked about his recent divorce. For some, sitting down next to a stranger on an airplane or train may produce a feeling of intimacy. It is safe to self-disclose to the person sitting next to you because you don't believe you will ever see him or her again. Sextimacy events can be similar to encountering a stranger on a plane in that proximity produces a sense of intimacy and not a history of shared experiences.

Physical intimacy mixed with self-disclosure is extremely compelling for women. You may find your sextimacy partner easily opens up about some aspects of his past or current life experiences, and yet, you have to remind yourself that there is no real closeness between you. This person knows nothing about who you are on a day-to-day basis, and you have no idea who he is. Becoming open and intimate is a gradual process that evolves over time, each layer of trust and acceptance building on the next. It is important to notice if in a short period of time you are either communicating a great deal of personal information to your sextimacy partner or if he is doing so. Although it may feel like real closeness, consider that it is more likely the joint effects of lust and not being in one another's day-to-day lives.

When the emotional intimacy you are experiencing with your partner is artificial, it may end quite abruptly. Nonetheless, women often remain feeling connected to sextimacy partners and attempt to rekindle feelings of closeness that seemed so intense early in the relationship. This is because women are driven to maintain and better their relationships and, as such, become emotionally invested. Research shows that women report they would feel more hurt by emotional infidelity (partner falling in love with someone else) than physical infidelity (one-night stand), while men report that physical infidelity would be more distressing to them.[18] The fear of losing the fantasy of possible, future emotional intimacy with a sextimacy partner can, at times, be so great that women maintain relationships with men who no longer meet their needs on any level.

THE EMPATHY TRAP

Women generally report experiencing greater empathy toward others than do men.[19] This begins in toddlerhood. Toddler girls seek to comfort those who experience distress and even stare more at others who are distressed than do toddler boys. The tendency of women to be more caring and empathic toward others holds true across a variety of cultures.[20] Empathic attunement is an enormous strength for women, as people who have a greater ability to understand the emotions of others have higher emotional intelligence and are better equipped to understand the motives of others.[21]

At the same time, experiencing empathy too intensely thwarts directly communicating one's own experience. Empathy for another can be so pronounced that you lose your connection with yourself and look at events from your partner's perspective more than from your own. A study found that women are more prone to experiencing guilt than men, and in particular, young women are susceptible to interpersonal guilt or guilt with regard to how one treats others in their life.[22] A prerequisite for experiencing guilt is having the capacity to deeply understand the feelings of others, or empathy. Women's hyper-socialization toward empathy results in many experiencing guilt needlessly. When women experience guilt, even when it is unwarranted, they tend to put their needs aside for those of their partner.

An example of how empathy can block communication is seen in the case of Sophie, who frequently argued with her romantic partner, Ryan, about feeling he was insensitive to her needs. On one occasion, Sophie arrived at a friend's party and found Ryan speaking intimately and cozily on the couch with another woman. Although Sophie smiled at him and tried to say hello, Ryan ignored her and eventually left the party without saying goodbye. Later that night, Ryan phoned wanting to meet. Sophie expressed irritation with Ryan for how he treated her at the party. Ryan responded with intense anger and defensiveness. He described having a difficult day, working too many hours, feeling mistreated by his boss, and feeling that Sophie was insensitive to his overall stress level. As he described his hardships, Sophie felt Ryan's anger intensifying and began to regret expressing her feelings to him at all. As Sophie described it, "I just kept thinking, I am too emotional, he just needs space, why do I always nag him? I just felt awful, like I was hurting him."

Sophie began to emotionally clean up the incident for Ryan; she spoke gently to him, offered apologies, and encouraged him to come over to her apartment. Sophie's feelings of irritation and hurt went unexpressed. Instead, Sophie put her energy into making Ryan feel better because, in her mind, she believed she upset him. Eventually Sophie learned that Ryan tended to turn the tables on her whenever she expressed any sort of complaint. Rather than soothing his upset, she learned to simply hear him out and then respond by repeating her original point, "I hear you, but you need to show me more respect."

It is important to notice when your empathy for the other person is blocking your ability to communicate your perspective. Stay with what you are feeling and observing. While listening to your partner, also work to not become overly caught up in the story of his experience; stick with your own perspective. I suggest to clients who particularly struggle with taking on the feelings of others to separate themselves from the situation: hang up the phone, go to the bathroom or a bedroom, and directly ask yourself what it is that is bothering *you*. Then find a way to put this into words. At times, you may need to continually repeat the same statement to your partner in order for him to hear you. The point is to not neglect your own perspective.

COMMUNICATE YOUR DRAMA

The goal in communicating your emotions is to find balance so that you neither avoid what you are feeling nor overwhelm others. Expressing emotion in a balanced manner fosters intimacy and closeness between romantic partners.

When you experience a negative emotion, there is frequently something that you need to communicate to someone in your life that may help you to feel better. When anger is felt, it often reflects the feeling that the self has been unfairly treated in some way. Once you have a sense of how you were unfairly treated, it may be helpful to respectfully put this into words and tell your partner so as to draw a boundary and clearly communicate your expectations of him. If you are feeling guilty about something and the guilt is reasonable given the situation, it can be relieving to make amends, tell the person you feel badly for the event, and apologize. When guilt is unwarranted, describe it to others so they may reassure you that you did not do anything wrong. When feeling sad, you may feel hopeless and alone in the world. The simple act of verbalizing sad feelings to another can help you feel more hopeful and connected.

As feelings are shared between partners, greater trust and acceptance develops. In order to build this trust, you have to initially be vulnerable and put your feelings into words to see how your partner responds. If, over time, you find your partner to be lacking in empathy and dismissive of your feelings, then this relationship may not be conducive to the intimacy you seek.

For real intimacy to develop, you need to be an effective listener when your partner communicates his emotional world to you. Don't lose yourself to empathy, but whether it be romantic partners or friends, learn to be gentle and not a hot poker in their emotional wounds. Act the way you wish to be treated when you are emotionally vulnerable. It is important both to do this for others and to choose companions who are able to do the same for you.

When conflict ensues in a relationship, people often feel their emotions at such an intense level that they become emotionally flooded. Emotional flooding is when your partner's behavior is entirely overwhelming. As described in the last chapter, when you are emotionally flooded, your amygdala has essentially taken over your cortex, and you are no longer able to think clearly. Communicating when emotionally flooded is ineffective and typically causes the conflict to escalate.

When emotionally overwhelmed, it is important to take time out and do one of the emotion-regulation strategies described in the last chapter, then come back to the person involved and talk more about what troubles you. Successfully managing conflict requires a balanced emotional state: If you feel too little emotion, you will not have the desire to resolve the conflict, and if you feel too much emotion, you may be unable to communicate effectively.

NEGOTIATE CONFLICT

Just as close relationships do not exist without conflict, close relationships do not flourish with unresolved conflict. Conflict tends to increase as people become more committed to one another, and it suggests the relationship is progressing in depth and importance to you. Experiencing conflict in a relationship is often a first step toward realizing you are becoming close to someone. The second step is to manage this conflict effectively. Conflict becomes torturous and intolerable when it is not managed through mutual communication and active listening to one another's grievances. When conflict goes unspoken, negative feelings are acted out through dysfunctional behavior, usually exacerbating the strife.

It is universal to want to avoid conflict. As a culture, we have developed all sorts of tactics to effectively avert directly voicing criticism that might provoke. These tactics include jokes or sarcastic comments to indirectly voice one's true feelings about another. Jokes and sarcasm generally have a hurtful edge. If you are on the receiving end and confront the other person, he or she may deny this edge by making you feel overly sensitive, saying, "Why are you so upset? I was just joking." Other tactics may include using a whiny voice, giving your partner dirty looks, angrily storming off and never telling your partner why, rolling your eyes, picking a fight while intoxicated, making your partner jealous through flirting with someone else, or giving your partner the silent treatment.

When these indirect methods are used to communicate negative emotion, your partner may have no idea what upset you. Because you are not explicitly stating what is bothersome to you, your partner may choose to deny, at least to himself, that he did anything wrong and thus avoid accountability. Women disempower themselves when they implement indirect means to express their angry or frustrated feelings. When you have the ability to clearly verbalize your feelings but choose to obfuscate, you sacrifice your self-respect and ability to get what you want in your relationships.

A typical way that unresolved conflict is managed in casual relationships is through a sort of cat-and-mouse game whereby one person (often the woman) makes demands as a way to deal with conflict, and the other person (typically the man) avoids conflict by changing the subject or leaving the scene. Women are generally the relationship managers who want change and, as such, are more likely to be in the demanding role. The person in the couple who is in the demanding role is typically the least powerful; as a result, she is usually unhappy with some aspect of the relationship. The person who is avoiding and withdrawing has the power and is getting his needs met in the relationship; he is safe in withdrawing because he is merely maintaining the status quo.[23]

This cat-and-mouse dynamic is often seen when the woman in a sextimacy relationship works hard to develop increased closeness from a withdrawn man who either lacks the desire or ability for emotional intimacy. The key aspect to this dynamic is that increased demands lead to more withdrawal, and more withdrawal leads to increased demands.[24] In the face of such adversity as withdrawn behavior and direct avoidance, some women continue to persevere in trying to connect. Ultimately this is self-defeating behavior—the more she works, the more he runs, and the more he runs, the more she works.

When a relationship is based on the cat-and-mouse dynamic, men often ratchet up their withdrawal tactic and avoid their partner when they want out of the relationship. Avoidance may range from completely severing all ties to just withdrawing subtly over time. This is an ineffective and immature communication strategy, but it does tell you a lot about the man.

Research shows that avoidance is the least effective and most upsetting way to end a relationship. Avoidance is indirect and, as such, can actually lengthen the breakup process because the other partner may believe she is not doing something quite right as opposed to understanding that the relationship is ending. Directly and mutually discussing the end of a relationship is the most effective way to move on.[25]

If you are the one ending a particular relationship, be straight and direct with your partner about why it will not work for you. If your partner is ending the relationship with you through avoidance, do not work to engage him once again; let him go and know that he is not for you.

It has been said time and again that couples should never go to bed angry. Going to bed angry actually is quite helpful in certain instances. As described in the previous chapter, when you experience intense negative emotion, it becomes difficult to discuss a conflict with a clear mind and with a voice that reflects your long-term goals. Taking time away from an argument may mean you have to leave the situation for a few moments, a few hours, or even for a day. If you decide to go to bed angry, it is essential that you not avoid the conflict entirely and revisit it sooner rather than later.

As you talk through your conflicts, adopt a collaborative framework where you are able to consider your partner's point of view without letting it override your perspective. Work toward a back-and-forth communication pattern where you listen, thoughtfully consider your partner's perspective, and then reconjure your own perspective and voice any discrepancies. This back-and-forth communication occurs over a number of cycles until the matter eventually resolves. When a relationship is healthy, couples are able to resolve the matter in such a way that makes both members feel better.

Some women tend to avoid this kind of back and forth because doing so brings them unnervingly close to their worst fear: rocking the boat and jeopardizing the viability of the relationship. This is why many women find themselves never bringing up what upsets them. Women who avoid conflict and go through their relationships with no voice have to make excuses to themselves in order to find ways to justify accepting men who do not fulfill them. Although harder in the moment, you are more likely to reach your longer-term goals of emotional closeness and satisfying relationships by learning to directly voice conflict in your relationships.

MIND READING

A well-known stereotype used against women is that they expect others, and in particular men, to read their minds. Women's cultural conditioning may make them prone to believing that others should intuit what they need or how they feel. Perhaps this is in part due to women's apt perceptive abilities. Many women are able to look at the people they love and, generally, have a sense of what they need or what they may be feeling. Women have perceptive abilities, but it is still impossible to accurately know one's innermost thoughts or feelings without direct verbalization. Although contrary to popular belief, the field of psychology is not at all based on the concept of mind reading. It is only through what other people say about themselves that you can begin to know who they are and what drives them at their core.

Many women do not directly communicate their negative feelings to others because doing so goes against their belief that likable girls get along and go along. For those women whose self-esteem is entirely rooted in others' positive appraisals of them, rocking the boat is feared and avoided at all costs. In fact, rocking the boat is so troubling that some women prefer to turn themselves inside out, morphing into whatever it is they believe others desire them to be. This is a doomed strategy, of course, as it means the woman never verbalizes her true self and so cannot partner with someone who is genuinely attracted to the real her. As described previously, even though one's thoughts or feelings may not be directly communicated, they often resurface in the form of relational aggression through gossip, manipulation, and generally passive aggressive behavior.

Certain emotions are typically more complicated for women to directly voice and are often acted out through self-defeating behavior. Jealousy, for example, is poisonous when not dealt with directly. Although many women refuse to talk about jealous feelings, research demonstrates that relational satisfaction actually increases when jealousy is discussed in an open and constructive manner. This may be because discussing jealous or insecure feelings frequently motivates a couple to revisit the boundaries of their relationship, and that revisit can strengthen their commitment to one another.[26] When you experience insecurity or jealousy, it is important to openly and honestly express your feelings.

This expression of genuine feelings, as opposed to seeing you flirt with another guy at a bar, will help your partner to understand you, and he will be less likely to view you as untrustworthy. On the other hand, if he cannot tolerate the expression of your genuine feelings, then you have learned much about his capacity for emotional intimacy. The problem is not the jealous feelings you may experience; it is how you choose to communicate them to your partner and how he receives them.

This is seen in the case of Caroline, a twenty-four-year-old graduate student who felt disappointed and continually let down by her sextimacy partner, Josh. She felt Josh did not spend enough time with her and that she was of little importance to him. Caroline gave Josh every clue to let him know how she felt, and she was fed up that he did not seem to get it. While out at a bar, she was frustrated and began to flirt with another guy in front of Josh. Josh became angry and flung a beer bottle at the man with whom Caroline was flirting. Josh and Caroline eventually left the bar together. The upheaval made Caroline feel as though Josh really cared about her. Caroline was again disappointed and defeated when, three days later, Josh chose to spend time with his friends instead of with her. She went back to flirting and working to make Josh jealous. Over time this behavior caused Josh to avoid Caroline altogether. In this way, Caroline created her worst fear and inadvertently encouraged Josh to disconnect from her.

An alternative way this could play out would be if Caroline had a conversation with Josh where she expressed something like the following: "I would like to spend more time with you, how do you feel about that?" Although a simple statement, it is direct and invites Josh to have a response. Listening to your partner's response is a key to knowing whether this is someone with whom you can become intimate. Whatever Josh may say is data about his ability to be emotionally intimate with Caroline. If he responds, "I would like that, too. Let's make that happen," that's great. If he says, "I do not want that kind of relationship right now," it's disappointing, but at least Caroline knows where she stands in the relationship. He may more likely say something in the middle, such as, "I would like that, too, but my schedule prevents that right now." This invites greater discussion, more negotiating, back-and-forth communication, and likely a few more conversations to get somewhere with the topic.

This back-and-forth process of eventually arriving at a resolution that meets both Caroline and Josh's needs is necessary for an emotionally close relationship to develop. If you do not directly state what you want, you do not give yourself the opportunity to learn where your partner stands in the relationship.

Research suggests that men actually want to communicate directly, and that it is women who, out of fear of what they might hear, tend to stop an open dialogue from occurring. Men are more likely than women to use direct strategies and open communication, while women are more likely to use pouting, hinting, or exhibiting a negative emotional state.[27]

When women use indirect communication strategies, it signals their lack of confidence and undermines their power in the relationship. If you rely on indirect communication strategies—whining, complaining, manipulating—you are ceding power in the relationship. Although these are all ways to communicate, directly stating your experience or preference is more effective, and women who directly communicate feel closer to their romantic partners.

Be direct, and tell your partners what you want. If you bclicvc your expectations are reasonable, and your partner either directly or indirectly lets you know that he cannot meet your needs or is unwilling to negotiate with you, move on. You avoid knowing the truth and settle for a relationship that is mediocre or worse by not stating your desires specifically. Instead of fearing his response, fear never asking the questions.

Challenge your thoughts about what it means to rock the boat—ask yourself, what is the worst-case consequence if you directly tell your partner how you feel? Ask yourself which of the following is in your long-term best interest: to never hear what you fear most from a romantic partner, or to hear it, grieve it, and move on. Choosing people with whom you can be sincerely yourself is one of the most liberating components of close friendship and intimate romantic partnership.

Be creative in terms of finding a medium that works. If a verbal, face-to-face conversation produces too much anxiety for you, use e-mail or text message. (One study found that adolescent girls are more likely to directly express their anger when they communicate through instant messaging than through direct face-to-face communication. When instant messaging with one another, teenage girls are more likely to use curse words, directly confront one another, and write about what bothers them.)[28] There can be missteps and mischief in the use of social media as well as in communicating face to face. The problem is not the tool but the way you use it. When it promotes a sincere and direct expression of feelings, social media is useful. The more you use direct communication, the more you will see that nothing terrible happens if you talk with people openly. As you learn to be direct, you will attract others in your life who are willing and able to hear you out and also willing and able to express themselves to you on a more intimate level.

USE POWERFUL SPEECH

To be direct and to be taken seriously by others, it is important to notice your voice tone and word choice. When women do express their desires directly, some compensate by using a passive, tentative, or apologetic tone. Research has shown that women are more likely to use powerless speech than are men, including questions that ensure the other person is on board with what they are saying: "Does that make sense?" or "Right?"[29] Appropriately soliciting the opinions of others is a valuable trait, but done mindlessly or compulsively, it becomes a block to effective communication. People who have less power or who hold lower status in a relationship are more likely to use powerless speech. The fact that women employ more powerless speech and indirect communication tactics than men reflects an imbalance of power that is present in many heterosexual relationships. Habitually utilizing powerless speech only serves to further disempower.

Some women also tend to nestle what they are saying in a thicket of apologies and disclaimers so that what they are attempting to communicate may not be fully detected. It is difficult to take someone's communications seriously when they are delivered with a weakened voice. Take these two statements, for example:

> "I am so sorry to bother you. I know you have a lot going on, but I just feel like we never see each other. I am sorry to be so annoying. I know how needy and overly emotional I can be."

Or

"I am feeling lonely in this relationship and would like to spend more time with you. Are you comfortable with the amount of time we spend together?"

The latter is an authentic representation of the speaker's feelings and invites further conversation so that she may understand more about where her partner is on this particular issue. Adopting empowering speech, along with solid eye contact, encourages others to listen to you, to respect you, and to take what you are saying seriously.

It is important to use a balanced voice when communicating, one that is not overly feminine or overly masculine in the traditional sense. When a man communicates with bravado, "Yo, where my dinner be?", he is not taken seriously by most. Likewise, if you voice your feelings in an overly feminine way out of a desire to remain nice, then what you are saying becomes wrapped in so much cotton candy that the listener just wants to move on to something more substantive.

CONCLUSION

In order for a mutually fulfilling and enduring relationship to develop, it is essential that you become comfortable in directly voicing your needs and preferences. Without expressing what you are feeling and thinking, you remain unknown to others. If you keep working at it, you will find a way to say just about anything. It may be difficult initially to find your voice, but what choice do you have? Is the threat of rocking the boat so terrifying that you are willing to settle for a serial disappointer and foreclose on your long-term happiness? Without question, when you are direct with people, some of your relationships will end. As hard as this may be, directly communicating with your partner forces you to hear the facts of the situation and to no longer make excuses for someone who does not have the strength of personality to meet your needs. Through directly stating your desires and upsets, you will find some of your relationships grow deeper and more intimate in ways you have never experienced. It is a risk worth taking.

SELF-ASSESSMENT: CAN YOU BE A CHATTERBOX WHEN YOU NEED TO BE?

Take this self-assessment to find out if you allow yourself to voice your emotions, thoughts, and experiences openly. The more yeses you endorse, the more prone you are to *not* rocking the boat. If you continually silence yourself, others do not know the real you, and you have no way to evaluate whether you can be emotionally intimate with your partners. The more items you endorse, the more you need to turn up the volume.

1. Certain topics are off limits with my partner.
2. I am careful to think about my partner's reaction to things before I discuss them.
3. I make sure not to ask my partner any question to which I do not wish to hear the answer.
4. I tell my friends about my upsets more so than my partner.
5. I try not to let my partner see me emote.
6. I am uncomfortable talking to my partner about my concerns in our relationship.
7. When my partner avoids a topic, I do not force the issue.
8. I am uncomfortable talking to my partner about the status of our relationship.
9. I do not ask my partner if he can commit to me.
10. I act like "one of the guys" around my partner so that he will feel comfortable with me.
11. When something bothers me in my relationship, I try to give my partner hints so that he will pick up on it.
12. I tend to avoid looking my partner in the eye and offer a lot of apologies when I upset him.
13. My partner and I are prone to extremes—either everything is peachy, or we are on the brink of destruction.
14. I prefer to let things run their course rather than openly discuss them.
15. I feel terribly guilty when I upset my partner.
16. When my partner upsets me, I do not return his calls, and I avoid him.

17. Sometimes I flirt with other guys to purposely make my partner jealous.
18. I tend to listen more to my partner's upset than express my own.
19. I usually feel as though things are fine with my partner, and then out of nowhere we will have a horrendous fight.
20. I only get into fights with my partner when I am intoxicated.

DECISION TREE: SHOULD YOU BRING UP AN ISSUE WITH A PARTNER?

This is a decision tree with items for you to consider when you are unsure whether it is in your best interest to bring up an issue or an upsetting event with your partner.

1. Are you ruminating a great deal about the issues, feeling anxious or experiencing muscle tension, headaches, or panic attacks?
2. Do you think about the issue a great deal or repeat it over and over again in your mind?
3. What will be the most likely outcome of talking about it?
4. What is the risk to you of talking about it?
5. How could you manage these risks should they occur?
6. What response are you avoiding by not talking about it?
7. What is the risk to you of not talking about it?
8. If you cannot speak directly to the person involved, is there anyone else who will listen and be compassionate and nonjudgmental?
9. Are you unhappy in your relationship with this person?
10. Do you feel inhibited when around your partner as a result of not communicating?

EXERCISES

The following are items to consider as you find your voice. It takes a bit of courage, but there is a way to say what needs to be said.

1. Is there anyone in your life that you can be straight with when they disappoint you? How are you different in this context? What is different about the relationship?
2. Talk with your significant others and close friends about wanting to be real and wanting them to be real; assure one another that direct communication does not have to lead to the ending of the relationship.
3. What are your fears in being direct with others about your negative feelings? Can you talk about these fears with those you are close to? Can you remind yourself that being direct may hurt in the moment but in the long run leads to more fulfilling relationships?
4. Practice broaching difficult topic areas with friends or partners. It can be helpful to begin difficult conversations by stating, "This is hard for me to say, and I want you to know I care about you, but . . . "
5. Role play with a friend different ways you could raise a difficult topic with your partner.

6

Dress Up

Developing Healthy Self-Esteem

Women who struggle with low self-esteem are at the mercy of others and utilize a coping strategy based on passivity. Low self-esteem and passivity are a toxic combination that accounts for why sextimacy relationships, and even abusive relationships, are endured over time. Many women admit to me with discomfort and embarrassment, "I have self-esteem issues," or "I just have never felt good about myself, even as a child." They are ashamed of these feelings and believe they are at fault. Some chronically replay negative thought streams on a daily or even hourly basis, each painful memory opening the door to another, producing a succession of pain. They tend to harshly judge and criticize themselves for this replay, thus triggering a new episode of negative thinking and despair. Feeling embarrassed by low self-esteem and at fault for the situation renders women powerless and unable to begin the process of finding their value separate from pleasing others.

In an effort to gain self-esteem, many young women turn to what they can control, developing and maintaining connections with others through focusing on the external. Popular culture promotes the idea that attractive women carry greater value and more easily develop relationships. Many women reduce feelings of disconnection and worthlessness by striving to appear more sexually desirable. Dressing up a negative self-image may mean new clothes, jewelry, a crash diet, or plastic surgery. In addition, low self-esteem leaves women vulnerable to sextimacy, as it too offers the possibility of the immediate rush of self-validation through temporarily connecting with another.

Self-esteem is not about self-perfection or about feeling superior to others. It is a process of learning to rebound from failures and disappointments with enough fortitude to hear criticism and consider feedback. Healthy self-esteem is striking a balance in which you accept yourself as you are while recognizing that with effort you can grow.

I recently saw a group of young girls, around eight or nine years of age, playing in the summer sun at a neighborhood park. They danced, lifted their shirts to cool themselves, laughed loudly, and shouted over one another to tell their own stories. They were genuinely full of themselves; they were all that and more. Learning to feel good about yourself is a return to this type of freedom. It is a return to individuality, spontaneity, and to the uninhibited ability to shamelessly bring yourself to life's table, however it may be set. The information provided in this chapter will help you lift the veil of anxiety and self-consciousness that contributes to low self-esteem.

THROUGH THE EYES OF OTHERS

Girls often sacrifice their independent discovery of who they are in order to live out the need to please others. In early childhood, girls are so good at the job of pleasing that they expect to hear they did a "good job" and are "perfect," "nice," "beautiful," "well-behaved," and "quiet." Research suggests that girls tend to hear these labels more than boys because girls are more emotionally mature and better behaved than boys in early childhood.

As they integrate these labels into their self-image, many girls pour everything they have into being perfect by way of grades, friendships, and meeting changing parental expectations. They relish the resulting accolades. By middle school and high school, life typically becomes more complicated as girls face demanding academics and relationships. With the added difficulty that life and school bring, girls begin to hear less that they are perfect, and as a result, their self-esteem may plummet.

Parents focused intensely on good or bad behavior, high or low grades, and strong or poor athletic abilities may miss the boat on teaching their girls how to manage adversity and setbacks. When challenges do surface, girls in particular become susceptible to anxiety and depression when they associate feeling challenged with not being good enough. If parents expect perfection and treat anything less with even mild criticism, girls who are ever aware of being judged learn to only feel worthwhile when they are hearing praise.

Carol Dweck, a professor and leading researcher in the area of social and developmental psychology, developed a theory of success that is based on extensive laboratory research. According to Dweck, people tend to develop a mindset or an internalized belief about what fosters their success. A fixed mindset is characterized by believing that we are born with a preordained amount of stuff—whether it is intelligence, personality, mood, athleticism, or sense of humor—and we either have these natural abilities or we do not. A fixed mindset is an all-or-nothing way of thinking about yourself—"Either I am a loser or a success," "Either I am a good person or a bad person," "Either I am desirable or undesirable."

Dweck found that praising children with labels such as "you are so smart" actually creates a fixed mindset and lowers IQ scores. Using all-or-nothing labels, such as "smart," "brilliant," or "beautiful," indirectly communicates to children that nothing will ever be a challenge because their innate abilities protect them. When they inevitably face difficulty or setbacks, self-esteem collapses, and fixed-mindset individuals tend to give up. According to Dweck, girls are more likely than boys to hold a fixed mindset (possibly due to the ways they are socialized) and so are less likely to take on challenges out of a fear of looking less than perfect.

On the other hand, a growth mindset acknowledges that we are born with certain temperamental and genetic propensities, but this mindset sees experience and learning as what really cause people to grow. While fixed-mindset individuals believe working at something means they are not smart/good enough, growth-mindset individuals believe effort and hard work pay off. When faced with negative feedback or when a flaw is exposed, growth-mindset individuals work harder and become more curious about finding an effective strategy.[1]

Here are statements, from Carol Dweck's *Mindset: The New Psychology of Success*, with which fixed-mindset individuals agree:[2]

> "You are a certain kind of person, and there is not much that can be done to really change that."
>
> "You can do things differently, but the important parts of who you are can't really be changed."

Here are statements that represent the growth mindset:

> "No matter what kind of a person you are, you can always change substantially."
>
> "You can always change basic things about the kind of person you are."

Failure is painful for growth-mindset individuals, too, but they tend to look at their setbacks as opportunities to learn and grow. Each relationship that does not work out and each goal that goes unreached are experienced as ways to gain useful feedback and develop as a person. This point of view helps maintain self-esteem even in the face of heartbreak and adversity.

Dweck researched individuals with depression and looked at their mindset. She found that both fixed- and growth-mindset individuals get depressed. As growth-mindset individuals felt more depressed, they actually took on greater responsibility to manage their problems; they worked even harder to take care of themselves and to keep up with their lives.

Fixed-mindset individuals feel shame and tend to give up when their shortcomings are exposed; for them, shortcomings mean they have a flaw that cannot be improved. Fixed-mindset individuals work hard to cover up their flaws. They are hyper-sensitive to perceived criticism and meet failures with defensiveness. For the fixed-mindset individual, self-esteem is entirely dependent on being right and perfect. They prove their worth by taking on low-risk experiences and relationships that do not challenge them.

When failure occurs, fixed-mindset individuals tend to fall apart. They face a flood of negative emotion that leaves no room to strategize or otherwise mitigate their circumstances. People who report that they are a "bad" person after a mistake are less inclined to seek forgiveness or repair the situation than people who feel that their behavior may have been "bad" but that they are not bad.[3] If you simply feel bad about your actions and not your entire character, then you are more likely to have the mental resources to repair the incident.

Many women do not learn as girls that they remain worthwhile even when they are not meeting the expectations of others. For these women, feelings of worthlessness take over when they receive criticism. What may just be a bad day turns into feeling like a bad person. These women are disconnected from an internal sense of fulfillment and only value themselves when others do.

"ALL THAT" GIRLS

In some social cliques, a woman who talks openly and confidently about her experiences ("I think I nailed that trig test" or "Ron is definitely asking me out tonight!") or who is not afraid to clearly state what she wants for herself ("Believe it, I am going to NYU") is labeled by members of the group as thinking she is "all that." Although girls are pressured at a young age to become all that, they also know that discussing their accomplishments makes other girls uncomfortable. In an effort to maintain the balance in their social group and to lessen envy or discomfort, some women do not discuss their happiest successes or innermost ambitions with other women.

Because many girls and women feel constrained by a straitjacket of having to be vigilant for their next big flop, they become anxious when they see another girl or woman openly speaking about the ways in which she feels positively about herself. The one speaking out may suddenly find that she is an outsider.

One of the implicit rules of being a "good girl" is that good girls do not act overly confident or show off their ambitions and successes because this violates the egalitarian structure of female relationships.[4] As Rachel Simmons, author of *Odd Girl Out*, observes, "The girl who thinks she's all that is the girl who expresses or projects an aura of assertiveness or self-confidence. She may assert her sexuality, her independence, her body, or her speech. She has appetite and desire. The girl who thinks she's all that is generally the one who resists the self-sacrifice and restraint that define 'good girls.' Her speech and body, even her clothes, suggest others are not foremost on her mind."[5]

The idea that a girl or woman may openly discuss herself in an unequivocally positive manner is threatening to those who are plagued by self-doubt and low self-esteem. Girls feel this tension with other girls, and when good things do happen to them, they typically shy away from outwardly praising themselves. They may communicate their accomplishments in a self-deprecating manner—"I guess I got lucky on that one."

Because women often have a refined capacity to intuitively feel the emotions of others, they know when they are making one another anxious and maintain a level of security in their relationships by not bringing too much of themselves to the fore. Even when they indisputably achieve a goal, many who suffer with low self-esteem are unable to fully appreciate their own accomplishments. They also have little experience in healthfully tolerating the accomplishments of their peers. Feelings of envy and competition are not managed directly and become compartmentalized, acted out indirectly through relational aggression.[6]

Talking enthusiastically about herself can make a woman dangerous to other women if it forces them to confront their own wish to be openly all that. Because of this tension, girls and women with low self-esteem are uncomfortable fully experiencing and communicating about their self-worth and ambitions. Instead, discussing negative self-perceptions is a dysfunctional way for these women to maintain their connections with other women.

WIRED FOR A NEGATIVE SELF-IMAGE

Genes and experience interact and make a lasting blueprint in the brain by influencing the ways synapses interact. How you know yourself on every level of your existence is represented within the wiring of your brain.[7]

The brain is comprised of billions of neurons that form trillions of synaptic connections. Chemicals are released, and electrical reactions are occurring continuously. Right now as you read this passage, billons of synapses are interacting and releasing chemicals so that your brain may encode the information. Neurons connect with one another in the brain through synapses, which allow chemical information to be exchanged and stored. When a neuron is in an active state, an electrical impulse travels down the nerve fiber and causes the release of a neurotransmitter from its terminal. The neurotransmitter is released into the synaptic cleft (the gap between the two neurons) and then binds to a dendrite on the receiving neuron, thus closing the gap between the two neurons. Most everything the brain does occurs through this process of neurons communicating with one another by synaptic transmission.

In his book *The Synaptic Self*, Joseph LeDoux draws on neurological research to explain how our sense of self is represented within our brains' neuronal wiring. As he describes it, "Nerve fibers are sort of like telephone wires. They allow neurons in one part of the brain to communicate with neurons in another. By way of these connections, communities of cells that work together to achieve a particular goal can be formed across space and time in the brain. This capacity underlies all of the brain's activities and is absent in other organs."[8]

Each time you are exposed to a similar life experience, the brain fires a specific pattern of neurons. Over time, familiar patterns of circuitry develop, which the brain effortlessly activates. Donald Hebb, a psychologist who worked extensively to understand the role of neurons in learning, developed a theory that explains how the brain changes as a result of new experiences. Hebb's influential theory is commonly referred to as "cells that fire together wire together." Hebb writes, "When an axon of cell A is near enough to excite cell B and repeatedly or persistently takes part in firing it, some growth process or metabolic change takes place in one or both cells such that A's efficiency, as one of the cells firing B, is increased."[9]

When new learning occurs, two neurons are active at the exact same time, and when the same learning experience occurs repeatedly, the two neurons develop a stronger connection and will fire more easily in the future. New learning experiences are remembered because they are sewn into the fabric of the mind by way of prior learning experiences.

A good example of new information becoming wired into the brain is seen in how young children learn language. For many toddlers, the first animal they see with regularity is the family dog. Consequently, when they first encounter another animal, say a cat, they may at first call it a dog because the neuronal wiring is already in place identifying that a furry, four-legged creature belongs to the dog neuronal network. In order to learn the various types of animals that exist, one must first learn that animals exist at all. The first animal sets up a blueprint in the brain that is embroidered and refined through experience over time.

How is all of this relevant for our purposes? Neuroscientists are now giving us a tangible, physical manifestation of why people get stuck in a downward spiral of low self-esteem and hopelessness. We all have a neuronal network for how we experience ourselves. We know how to view ourselves as a result of this network. True to reality or not, it tells us if we are capable, lovable, and effective.

The brain works each new experience into its memory by fitting it into the preexisting neuronal pattern. If early on in your development your parents, teachers, and peers were regularly critical and judgmental of you and did not attend to your needs or feelings, then your sense of self may be based on feeling unworthy and unlovable. Perhaps as a child each time you failed at a task or became emotionally distraught, your parents responded with "You should have studied harder" or "You need to lose weight, then the other kids will like you" or "Stop being a drama queen." Perhaps in your childhood you moved a great deal, and each time you entered a new school you were made fun of or felt different from your peers. Or you may have struggled with a learning disorder or a medical condition that set you apart, so you felt different or less than others. With repeated experiences of mistreatment, a negative self-image becomes a well-worn neuronal pathway.

Each time you have a setback or feel vulnerable, your brain will call up this negative self-image and trigger a series of roughly similar thoughts or memories that remind you of your every shortcoming. You may not like this or even consciously want it, but due to your past experiences of repeated mistreatment or alienation, your brain is wired for a negative self-image.

If you suffer from low self-esteem, when good things do happen to you, it may be hard to fully take in the experience because positive experiences do not match your well-worn neuronal circuitry. Your brain is conditioned to make you feel poorly about yourself simply because this pattern is familiar and requires no effort. In order for your brain to expend the least energy possible, it repeatedly triggers this familiar, and thus easy, negative self-image circuitry. It will direct you to your flaws as well as partners and experiences that confirm your negative self-image.

When the model for one's self-image is negative, the neuronal networks will continue to fire down the same old road of self-doubt and self-criticism. Each new negative thought brings to mind negative thoughts from the past and keeps you in a circular trap.[10] Indeed, for many, these negative thought streams have fired for so long that they are cued without a person's conscious awareness.

HOW TO REWIRE AND BECOME UNSTUCK

For many years neuroscientists believed that by the age of two, human brains have all of the neurons that they will ever have. Current research is showing that new neurons (neurogenesis) can grow in parts of the hippocampus (the brain's memory storehouse) in healthy adult brains. New experiences change our neuronal wiring through a chemical process termed long-term potentiation (LTP). LTP is the actual chemical mechanism through which learning and memory occur in the brain.

In laboratory experiments, researchers have found that LTP of a neuronal pathway (through rapid electrical stimulation) caused a stronger synaptic response in this pathway later, when compared to baseline measures.[11] In other words, if a person repeatedly engages a new experience (thus continually firing the same neuronal pathway), the new experience becomes part of the person's brain system on a chemical level.

A real-life example of this would be if you decided to learn to speak French. You are unlikely to learn the language if all you do is periodically study a few vocabulary words. On the other hand, if you live in France with a French family, work in a French company, and force yourself to speak French all the time, you will likely repeat French language experiences often enough to begin to actually learn French.

Studies conducted on orphans from World War II and the Korean and Romanian conflicts demonstrate the profound impact that new experience can have on the brain's wiring. Many of these children had no attachment to a caretaker. At the time they were adopted, these orphans were often emotionally regressed and physically emaciated. After several years of healthy family life with their adoptive parents, most of these children were psychologically well adjusted and demonstrated improved cognitive functioning.[12]

The research unequivocally shows that the brain can adjust and adapt through neuronal plasticity. Athletes, musicians, and meditative monks have increased their brains' capacity for their specialized pursuits. Individuals who lose the ability to see or to hear develop increased neuronal connections for their other senses; for example, the deaf often have heightened peripheral visual attention.[13] Working over and over again at something new physically changes the brain's wiring.

The synaptic pathways involved in attention, thinking, mood, motivation, and emotional regulation can all be altered by new learning through life experience. The process through which one develops low self-esteem (repeatedly feeling criticized and undervalued) is the same process that may undo a negative self-image (repeatedly engaging new experiences that provide positive feelings). Psychotherapy is an excellent example of a new learning experience that changes brain wiring; ideally each week when you encounter your therapist, you develop a more positive experience of yourself. As this occurs repeatedly over time, neurological research suggests that therapy rewires the brain through changing synaptic connections.[14]

If you suffer from chronic low self-esteem, it is likely you are harboring certain schemas about yourself that are ineffective or toxic but reflect well-worn patterns of synaptic activity. Just like a song you cannot get out of your head, negative thought streams will replay unless you provide your brain with new experiences. You have a choice in terms of whether you will allow a new experience to take hold in your mind or continue down the same old negative thought stream. As Joseph LeDoux observes, "That the self is synaptic can be a curse—it doesn't take much to break it apart. But it is also a blessing, as there are always new connections waiting to be made."[15] When you engage new learning experiences and repeatedly activate more positive associations of thought, your neuronal circuitry will change, and even when you feel defeated or disappointed, it will be easier to cue a positive thought stream.

JUST DON'T *WANT* TO DO IT . . .

Have you ever had the experience of knowing you should do something but having no desire to do it? Perhaps you know that going to the gym, calling a friend, or completing a work assignment will make you feel better about yourself, and yet, you just can't get yourself to act. Maybe you even know that doing the strategies discussed in this chapter will help you to feel better about yourself, and yet, you have no motivation to do so. This occurs because, as described in the last chapter, the brain is not an equal opportunity connector. Higher-order thinking systems do not have strong connective wiring to the more primitive emotional brain. The brain has a slight disconnect between thinking and feeling; we may know something to be true and, simultaneously, lack the emotional motivation to do what needs to be done.

Thinking overrides our more primitive base needs all the time, but this does not occur automatically and does require significant effort. People stop smoking, stop drinking, begin exercising, become parents, quit cheating, become religious, become vegetarian, and undertake any number of other life-altering initiatives. People change all the time. We all have the capacity to do so. It is a matter of putting in the effort. Particularly when trying to develop a new behavior or outlook, you may have to force yourself to go through the motions again and again for months at a time, but you will eventually feel the rewards of your work.

If you keep thinking and experiencing what you have always thought and experienced, the brain's wiring will remain the same. If you allow it to do so, the brain has an extraordinary ability to adapt and grow in the face of new experience. The remainder of the chapter addresses new approaches and behaviors that, when used with regularity, will reset your self-perception.

REDUCE STRESS

Neuronal growth occurs in our brains when we learn new information, but new growth actually decreases when we are in a distressed state.[16] The hippocampus (the brain's memory storehouse) is dependent on glucose for energy. Stress hormones decrease glucose in the brain and thus render the hippocampus less effective. In order to learn and to fully take in new experiences, possibly even grow new neurons, and certainly change synaptic connections, stress must be reduced. If you engage in new experiences while experiencing anxiety, worry, or repetitive negative thoughts, the new experience will not effectively imprint in the memory storehouse.

Adopt a daily relaxation ritual to lessen anxiety and calm the brain. Examples of relaxation exercises that work effectively to reduce stress include meditation, yoga, guided visualization, mindfulness, acupuncture, massage, and breathing exercises. It is important to find an exercise that works well for you and to practice it regularly, even if only for a few minutes.

SHINE THE SPOTLIGHT WHERE IT COUNTS

You want to focus your attention like a spotlight on your goals and hopes for the future, not on your flaws and past failures. If you struggle with low self-esteem, then you are perpetuating your negative sense of self through repeating the same dysfunctional thought streams. It is important to notice the content of your thoughts so they do not play unchallenged. Consider what thought streams, memory sequences, or negative events tend to repeat.

As you begin to consciously observe your thought stream, notice how each thought influences the next. Perhaps you have a hard day at work or feel your boss doesn't value you, and then you flash back in time to an old boyfriend who made you feel worthless, and you begin to remember the painful things he said. By the end of this thought cycle, you are likely going to feel even worse about your day. As you gain greater conscious awareness of your thoughts, it will be easier to pull out of a negative thinking spiral and engage in the present moment.

Notice when you are caught in a negative cycle, and redirect your attention to the present moment. If you are working, work to the best of your ability; if you are talking with a friend, attend to her every word; if you are on a date, bring your entire self to the occasion. There will be hurdles—your mood at that time, your energy level, other events in your life, your health. The goal is to do the best job you possibly can in that moment.

If you find you continue to ruminate or think critically about yourself, schedule a set time to worry and be self-critical—2:00 to 2:20 p.m. on Friday, only focus on worrying and cut yourself off when the allotted time has elapsed. People who schedule time to put all of their attention into worrying report that they actually run out of things to think about during the allotted time and worry less at other times of the day.

BECOME YOUR OWN BEST CARETAKER

In order to maintain a sense of control and internal contentment separate from your relationships with others, it is important to adopt a healthy lifestyle. It seems simple, but the fact is too many people, particularly those with low self-esteem, neglect the basics of self-care. The goal is not to become obsessive about your health routine but to develop a solid balance.

Imagine your relationship with yourself as similar to how you would treat a small child entrusted to your care. Would you berate the child and remind her of her every imperfection or past mistake? As she enjoys her friends or engages in a homework assignment, would you pull her attention away and remind her of how she blew it with her last best friend or did poorly on a recent school exam? Would you allow a child in your care to stay up all night and eat junk food, day after day? Would you encourage a child in your care to starve herself so as not to become fat? Would you speak harshly and abusively toward the child?

When those with low self-esteem consider these questions, they report that they would take better care of a child than they do themselves. Children benefit from a daily routine that includes nutritious food, a bit of exercise, a stimulating activity each day, and kindness; adults sometimes forget that they need the same.

One of the most powerful ways to increase the happy chemicals in the brain is through exercise. Develop a realistic exercise plan you can stick to consistently. The point is not to run the Boston marathon (unless you want to!) but to develop a routine that matches your ability and desires. Your goal may be to walk four miles. You simply begin walking until you feel fatigued, then stop and start again the next day, gradually building up to four miles. Eating a balanced and nutritious diet also helps to keep your mood and energy in check. Finally, it is helpful to set aside time each week to manage the regular upkeep of your life—bills, house cleaning, grocery shopping, work assignments. If you allow these tasks to pile up, then you will repeatedly remind yourself of what you have not done and fill yourself with dread.

You do not need to eat healthfully, exercise, and attend to your life tasks in an obsessive manner. Simply keep a general routine for more days than not. Part of being your own best caretaker is allowing yourself to indulge.

It is empowering to take control of your happiness through developing a simple daily routine that puts you in the driver's seat of your life. Recognize that it is self-destructive not to allow yourself to do these simple things.

CHANGE YOUR APPROACH TO SETBACKS

When you feel as though your successes and failures are a statement of your worth, challenges are particularly intimidating because too much of your self-worth is at stake. On the other hand, self-esteem skyrockets when you cultivate goals based on your innermost desires and when you develop a belief that persistence will enable you to actualize these goals. Social science research shows that when people are told that hard work and effort improve performance, IQ and academic scores actually improve.

At the end of this chapter, you will find a self-assessment that will help you to determine if you allow yourself to grow from your mistakes or if your mistakes signify to you an inescapable character flaw. It is important when assessing your approach to setbacks to notice your internal narrative. Your internal narrative is the voice in your head that is commenting on what you are experiencing in the world. Notice what the voice is saying when you experience failure or receive negative feedback. Is there kindness in your internal voice, or is it a punitive voice? Notice the tone of your voice. Is it harsh and angry or soft and compassionate?

Just as test scores are improved by studying, so too can self-esteem scores be improved with practice. Remind yourself that effort pays off; notice when you are punishing yourself for a perceived defect. Find a way to see yourself as a work in progress. When you want to give up in your pursuit of feeling better about yourself, continue to work at it despite doubts or second thoughts.

Each time you challenge yourself with experiences that do not come easily, you are increasing the strength of your brain on a neuronal level. Stop avoiding people and events that foster feelings of insecurity. Intentionally seek experiences that are hard for you so you may learn to become comfortable with them. Surround yourself with people who challenge you intellectually, romantically, and emotionally.

Learn to take on professional and social ventures even when they make you feel uncomfortable so that you may find new strategies for managing them. If you struggle with communicating your needs or managing conflict in relationships with men, then each relationship is an opportunity to work on improving these skills. Stop avoiding what scares you or makes you doubt yourself. Build a positive experience of yourself confronting what does not come easily. The way you feel can be improved by trying new things.

As you give up your preoccupation with self-criticism, your mind will have more resources to actually learn from the difficult situations you encounter. Setbacks are hard but easier to manage when you remember that you will be enriched by your challenges, as long as you choose to view them as avenues for growth.

STAY CONNECTED WITH YOURSELF

Many women tell me that relationships are their Achilles' heel. Although they are smart, have interesting jobs, or may be attending good universities, every time they are within the presence of an attractive man who is interested in them, they yield. Wanting affection from a man trumps the need to assess whether he will make a healthy partner. The woman too often focuses her attention on whether or not the man is responding favorably to her. She becomes so enraptured by feeling his affection and validation that she does not stop to assess whether he is a suitable match. She is so needy for the affection and temporary intimacy that there is no space to consider the man from the perspective of her best long-term interest. Rather than making a conscious assessment, she spends her time obsessing about her flaws and ruminating about what he may or may not think of her.

In order to feel better about yourself and enjoy your life to the fullest, it is essential that you have a separate sense of self. If your sense of self-worth depends on how other people treat you, then you do not have a separate sense of self.

When you have low self-esteem, you may suffer from what I call the sponge effect. The sponge effect is a tendency to soak up the negative emotions of others or to take on excess responsibility to please others. In a study that asked college students to interpret an ambiguous message about the reason a potential romantic partner was unable to spend time with them, the results suggested that college students with low self-esteem were more likely to report blaming themselves for the rejection than those without low self-esteem.[17] In order to build your sense of self, recognize when you are becoming a sponge or are tending to the perspectives of others. Instead of focusing on what is going on for others, tune into what is going on for you.

Work to see how you experience yourself through your own eyes: What do you like, what do you dislike, what do you need, how do you feel with various people and in various settings? Turn down the volume on other people's feelings, needs, and desires, and stay connected with yourself. Notice when you are imagining what someone else might think of you and redirect your attention spotlight to what *you* think of you. Observe when you feel a sense of internal peace, even if it is fleeting, or when you feel displeasure. When you have ambivalence, this is often a signal that you are disconnected from yourself. Rather than just going forth, sit down and try to explore what your feelings or needs are in the situations you encounter.

Another way to stay connected with yourself is by consciously listening to your internal narrative. Again, your internal narrative is that little voice in your head that is commenting and making observations about whatever it is you are experiencing in that moment. For some, the voice has been dulled, invalidated, and put in its place for so long that they may no longer have full access to it. It is essential that you begin to excavate your internal narrative and notice how it serves to help or to hinder you. Notice if the voice in your head speaks to you with a judgmental or angry tone and how this tends to add to your insecurities and tension. Consider softening the tone and making the voice speak in a way that is more supportive of your goals.

The importance of learning to become more connected with yourself is seen in the case of Chelsea. Chelsea had a long history of difficulty with relationships and a pattern of using men for her sorely lacking sense of self-validation. When she was in a social situation, she worked double time to assess what she thought the object of her desire would be attracted to and then to act the part. If he liked funny, she became a comedian; if he liked intellectual, she scrutinized the Sunday paper; if he was into sports, she took on his favorite team. If a partner became upset about anything, she felt guilty and frantically worked to make him feel better. She never felt secure about her body and painstakingly worked to camouflage her perceived flaws.

As she participated in therapy, Chelsea became more aware that her internal voice was judgmental and punitive. When around a guy she was interested in, her voice would say, "You better not eat that burger. He is going to know you are a pig," or "Don't turn around, or he will see how big your ass is," or "He is upset, what have you done now?" or "Be funnier. You are so boring, why would anyone want to hang out with you?"

Chelsea came to see how much she mistreated and abused herself in social settings. She learned to use a softer tone and to be accepting and compassionate with herself. Most importantly, she trained her voice to support her goal of living in the present and gaining greater pleasure from her life.

After a trip to the beach with some male and female friends, Chelsea came into my office exuberant. She had the time of her life and not because of a hookup. The highlight from her trip was jumping in and out of the ocean with abandon. In the past, when she went to the beach, her entire goal was to keep her stomach pulled in tight. She would force herself into a fixed position on the beach and move as little as possible so as not to expose physical flaws. This trip, however, she successfully distracted from thoughts related to body image and appearing sexually pleasing to men. When her internal dialogue was no longer obsessed with retaining the perfect pose, Chelsea noticed that the little voice in her head wanted her to jump in the water and swim. By working to stay connected with this desire, Chelsea acted on it and went in and out of the ocean without self-consciousness and with much delight.

STOP "HATING ON" YOURSELF

Women cripple themselves with astonishing frequency through harsh self-criticism of their physical appearance. Many of the women I talk to refer to this act quite casually: "I was hating on myself all night." Hating on oneself means repeatedly picking apart every perceived physical concern imaginable. They hate on themselves with little conscious awareness of this pernicious, emotionally debilitating inclination.

Develop self-awareness for when you are entering hating-on-yourself territory and evacuate immediately. Take a cold shower, go for a jog, or call a friend, but you need immediate distraction. Every time you allow this self-abuse to take over your thinking, you are discarding your self-worth.

With regard to physical appearance, it can be helpful to remind yourself that the ideal female body type is not fixed but changes over time. Once a heavier body was considered healthier, and thus sexier, while a thin body was associated with the inability to conceive a child and, as such, was seen as weak and unattractive. Also, when getting enough to eat is a struggle for a society in general, weight may become a status symbol signaling an enviable access to extra calories. For some, Marilyn Monroe, curvaceous and distinctly not anorexic, set a standard for sexual attractiveness in the late 1940s and 1950s. Over time that standard began to give way to Twiggy's thin and somewhat androgynous look. That was followed by thin waifs with enormous breasts, a combination not often found in nature but achieved routinely with breast implants. The point is, the popular look changes. Women often feel the need to adapt to this changing standard, which is usually set by men. Self-interest is better served when you set the standard for yourself.

WELL-ADJUSTED FEMALE FRIENDS

Relationships are a sacred part of our existence; they enable us to endure life's stressors and to find greater meaning. Healthy friendships are your armor, making you less likely to hate on yourself and need sextimacy for self-validation. Women have a special ability to form connections and get close to others; use this strength intelligently by picking nonjudgmental, accepting friends.

It is a disconcerting but well-known truth that women often have certain, vague fears about one another that go unexamined. Frequently in my work with women, when I suggest that they open up to a friend about a problem they are having, they give me a knowing look and say, "You know how women can be," implying that other women cannot be trusted and are deeply petty. If you harbor these types of beliefs about your own sex, it is time you begin to challenge where they come from. Women who align themselves in healthy friendship, encircled with safety and trust, are likely to excel on every level. Dating, motherhood, academic pursuits, new jobs, illness, grief, and more all become significantly easier to endure with the support of a strong group of women.

Treat other women the way you wish to be treated. Work to build a safe harbor, where trust and openness permeate. Leave judgment at the door, and foster empathy. You will promote a deep sense of closeness and comfort by allowing your friends to talk and by listening carefully to them.

There is no age limit on friendship; younger women and older women remind us of where we have been and where we are going. Find women who nurture and guide you and for whom you do the same. Find women with whom you can unabashedly celebrate your accomplishments.

Look for friends who are as good to you as you are to them. You cannot care for others more than you care for yourself; when someone makes you feel badly on a consistent basis, consider talking with her about it. If she can hear your feelings and you agree to work on the issue, then continue the friendship. If your friend cannot hear you out and consistently treats you in a manner that makes you feel unhappy, consider ending the friendship. It is okay not to be close to everyone who will have you, so pick wisely.

THE ILLUSION OF FUSION

There is a danger in being too dependent on others. Socialization encourages young girls to attend to others more than to themselves, and by womanhood, identity is sometimes fused to relationships.[18] Women can become so inherently tied to people that it becomes hard to retain a separate sense of self. Many do not know themselves outside of being someone's daughter, mother, friend, or lover. When this is the case, self-esteem may depend almost completely on those relationships.

Women who experience self-worth only in the context of relationships are more vulnerable to sticking with partners and friends who are harmful. Those who are entirely dependent on relationships for their sense of adequacy struggle with effectively facing the world alone. For some women, being alone means unbearable feelings of emptiness. Sextimacy is a balm for these feelings. But whatever the level of relief, it is felt temporarily and usually comes at the price of submitting to an utterly one-sided relationship.

Develop a tolerance for yourself on your own, without others around. If you can't stand to be with yourself alone, then how will anyone else stand to be with you? Learn to be alone through meditating each day about your goals for yourself; bring your full intention to the picture as you visualize exactly what you want to feel inside and what you want to be doing on the outside. Picture your life going the way you want it to go; imagine obstacles and challenges, but in your imagination, find ways around these challenges. Limit the time spent feeling badly about yourself when something does not work out. Sit quietly, and imagine the same event happening but unfolding the way you wish.

It is possible to fill emotional voids by being in a constant state of action and by feeling busy and stressed. Perpetual action is a diversion. Perhaps you go from one social event to the next, work long hours, and constantly have activities to fill your spare time. When you do have a moment alone, you feel uncomfortable and immediately find ways to busy yourself. If you do not make time for yourself to thoughtfully consider what you want, what you want can never come. You and only you are in control of your life. If you are too busy to spend time with yourself, you are undervaluing yourself, and you will choose partners who treat you similarly.

Ask yourself what are you avoiding by being so busy. Are you afraid of quiet time? What is the hardest part for you about being alone? Remember what you learned in chapter 4 about how emotions work. Allow your emotions to come in and be felt. Accept those feelings. See if you can learn something new about yourself simply by being quiet and feeling whatever may come up for you when alone.

Find aspects of your identity to hold on to that are separate from your relationships with others. As Freud aptly observed a century ago, work and pleasure make for a balanced and contented life. Allow yourself to consider what it is that may satisfy your thinking self. Whenever a relationship is not going smoothly, you can turn to your work or other interests for needed validation and meaning. Broaden your image of yourself. Those women who occupy more diverse roles—for example, daughter, student, musician, and political volunteer—often feel more positively about themselves.

Professional endeavors, artistic pursuits, developing one's spirituality, taking an interest in politics, and pursuing intellectual interests all contribute to a positive sense of self. Develop control over your compulsion to be pleasing to others and put this energy into developing your interests and forming a lasting sense of connection with the world around you. You no longer need to be a lady-in-waiting for Mr. Right to make you feel good. You have the power to make yourself feel good.

SEXTIMACY AND LOW SELF-ESTEEM

If you struggle with chronic sextimacy and have difficulty forming relationships with partners who are consistently loving toward you, your brain may have developed an association early in life that loving others is linked with disappointment and feelings of unworthiness. Children are cognitively unable to objectively recognize their parents' weaknesses. When they are let down by their parents or emotionally neglected, children believe they caused their parents' inept behavior and adopt a mindset of "If they don't like me, then I don't like me either." When treated poorly, children feel worthless and flawed and believe that if they were not flawed, their parents would take better care of them. As adults, they continue to harbor the belief that they are not sufficiently worthwhile to sustain a loving relationship.

Feeling unworthy and rejected is painful, and this pain causes an urgent desire to repair the damaged self, setting the stage for sextimacy, which further perpetuates a lack of self-regard. This circle is not the path to sexual fulfillment and emotional intimacy.

Many struggling with low self-esteem tell me they are not attracted to men who directly state their desire to date them. I ask these women, why not? They tell me they want a challenge, or they say they believe men who express their intentions are somehow soft or not as masculine. They may list various *Seinfeld*-like quirks that they just cannot tolerate—"It's the way he chews his food," or "His mother called during our date." Whatever they say, what these women mean is they cannot be attracted to someone who directly communicates an interest in them. For women who struggle with sextimacy, nice guys do not match their neuronal wiring for a negative self-image, and as such, it feels odd, uncomfortable, and burdensome to become romantic with men who directly and positively pursue them.

As long as you view yourself as not good enough, you will choose partners who replay this negative self-image. Your neuronal pattern screens out those who see you more positively than you see yourself. If you do not work on feeling better about yourself, you will continue to develop relationships with men who are arrogant and never pleased by you.

If you struggle with sextimacy, you need an exercise regime to build your self-esteem. Just like lifting weights for the first time, start with light weights and build up from there. Little by little you will change your brain's wiring every time you talk about or directly experience men who treat you well. Overcoming sextimacy means confronting your negative self-image and beginning to work on becoming the person you wish to be. By no longer allowing yourself to seek quick-fix solutions, including sextimacy, you give yourself an opportunity to form a healthy relationship with yourself and a permanent sense of contentment.

CONCLUSION

Negative thoughts can be turned around quickly if you allow yourself to have other experiences that make you feel good and remind you of what matters most in the world to you. Recognize that a moment of feeling flawed does not have to translate into a lifetime of feeling not good enough. As you fully participate in your life, the paralysis induced by low self-esteem will fade.

You are not at the mercy of life. You control your actions and reactions. If you treat yourself with acceptance and challenge yourself to grow, you will develop a sturdy sense of self that will rebound from setbacks. As it eventually becomes second nature for you to value yourself in this way, you will find you are attracted to healthier partners who confirm your positive self-image. The final chapters explore how to begin applying your emotional awareness, direct communication, and your growing self-esteem to your romantic relationships.

SELF-ASSESSMENT: DETERMINE YOUR LIFE APPROACH

Take this self-assessment[19] to find out if you allow yourself to grow from your mistakes or if your mistakes signify to you that you are impossibly flawed. More yeses suggest you are prone to not allowing yourself to evolve to become the person you wish to be. If you continually gauge your worth by how others see you, your self-esteem will remain fragile.

1. When I hit a setback, I doubt myself and often give up.
2. When something doesn't work out for me, I beat myself up with criticism.
3. Even when I do achieve a goal, I immediately begin to feel anxious about the next task on my list.
4. Most of what I do is to prove my worth to others and less about what I desire.
5. When I sense that someone is about to give me negative feedback, I withdraw, change the subject, or become defensive.
6. I do not believe that I can grow from my mistakes.
7. I want to stay just as I am, but I am unhappy where I am.
8. Sometimes after a social event I feel great about myself, but within a few hours or a day, I feel depleted.
9. I am worried that people will see me as a fraud, and I will be exposed.
10. I do not believe that the aspects of my personality that bother me are changeable through learning and new experience.

7

Kissing a Frog

Dating with Self-Awareness

In order to develop your identity in your romantic relationships, live as though you already know how the storyline of your romantic life unfolds. Believe with every fiber of your being that not only will you find your Prince Charming, but you will also be happier than you imagined possible, and that you will likewise be fine being alone for periods of time, even if finding a life-mate is your goal. Instead of being consumed by anxiety and fear of a life alone, embrace dating as a self-discovery process. Dating experience teaches you who you are in relationships and what fulfills you. You may learn the most in this regard from those connections that do not lead to permanent commitment. In the fairy tale, when the princess kissed the frog, the frog turned into her Prince Charming. But, as you know, it does not always work that way—sometimes you discover you are kissing a frog that does not change into anything at all. The fact that you kissed a frog is not a statement of your worth but, rather, part of your education. This education will eventually lead to a mutually loving, satisfying relationship.

In the list of things that may influence how we see ourselves, little compares to the impact of those with whom we choose to become close. Intimate relationships are so rewarding that in certain settings, just being in the presence of those you cherish will leave your brain awash in endorphins. The loss of love or the lack of love in one's life brings tremendous pain and suffering. In their book *A General Theory of Love,* three psychiatry professors, Thomas Lewis, Fari Amini, and Richard Lannon, use the newest scientific discoveries in brain research to explain how our nervous systems are innately wired for intimacy and human connection. As they state, "We are attached to keep our brains on track, in a process that begins before birth and sustains life until its end."[1]

We need one another in order to stay grounded in the here and now and to give life meaning. When isolated, people report feeling anxious, obsessive, disoriented, and depressed. The need to feel less alone in the world is so primal that when healthy prospects are absent, people will partner with the unhealthy. Developing healthy connections is essential for your wellbeing and contentment. Unhealthy relationships filled with tension and stress decrease life satisfaction, lower immunological functioning, decrease resiliency to stress, and may lead to a shorter lifespan.[2]

In the previous three chapters, we explored the importance of developing greater intimacy with yourself through learning to understand and manage your emotional world, forming a strong voice reflective of your needs and desires, and building your core self-esteem. Building this core sense of self and self-acceptance is essential to developing emotionally intimate relationships with others. In this chapter, we will explore your history with love and how to build a new, more fulfilling love pattern. You will develop a road map showing where to travel romantically and what spots to avoid by understanding your experience in relationships, including with whom you choose to become intimate, and how you may avoid repeating certain dysfunctional dynamics from your past.

LOVE HISTORY

Mary Ainsworth and her colleagues demonstrated in revelatory attachment research that newborn babies come equipped with a whole series of "proximity promoting" behaviors. Moments after birth, newborns grasp their caregiver's finger or sleep more easily when pressed against the warmth of another. Babies use their attachment repertoire—cooing, crying, gazing, cuddling, and crawling—to bring people closer.

All of these behaviors elicit care and nurturing from others and encourage connection.

Exactly how effective parents are in attaching with their children creates big differences in how their children achieve a healthy self/other balance.[3] Attachment with caretakers informs a child, as each emotion or need experienced is mirrored in her parents' faces. If hungry, the child is presented food. If sad, the child is soothed. Needs are eased with parental responsiveness. If attachment to caregivers goes well, brain growth flourishes, and the child learns the world is a safe place where relationships offer comfort and a sense of wellbeing.

The authors of *A General Theory of Love* use the term "limbic resonance" to describe humans' amazing way of connecting with one another emotionally: "A symphony of mutual exchange and internal adaptation whereby two mammals become attuned to each other's inner states."[4] Limbic resonance is the process through which two nervous systems connect, so they come to intuitively understand and care about one another's circumstance. This emotional synchrony is seen when observing mothers and babies, intimate lovers, and close friends. Limbic resonance is so powerful that our relationships with others have the potential to calm distress and even to rewire the brain's expectations about love and relationships. "The timeworn mechanisms of emotion allow two human beings to receive the contents of each other's minds. Emotion is the messenger of love; it is the vehicle that carries every signal from one brimming heart to another. For human beings, feeling deeply is synonymous with being alive."[5]

Responsive and tender caretakers are skilled in reading their children's emotional cues. Through time, the back-and-forth process of emotional empathy in childhood becomes internalized so that in adulthood, people are able to make themselves feel better when distressed and more easily choose mates who share a similar relationship wiring.

When one or both caretakers are unpredictably responsive to their child's needs, consistently distracted, or inattentive, they may leave children with an insecure love history. Because they were not given adequate emotional nurturance as children, adults with a history of insecure attachment have difficulty understanding their emotions and difficulty reassuring themselves when things go wrong. Adults who have a history of insecure love do not expect relationships to consistently bring comfort and tend to pick partners who confirm their brain's wiring for a negative self-image.

If you have experienced a problematic love pattern in your history then you may be drawn into relationships with partners who are inconsistent in their love for you, partners who are aloof and disinterested in knowing the real you. Your relationships may have sporadic periods of closeness followed by distance and despair.

Just as it is true for the child, adult love involves a foundation of trust and a sense of emotional comfort, both of which help the adult take on new challenges. What once was a son hearing his mother encourage him to take his first steps turns into a spouse telling his wife, "Go for it, you can get that promotion," or "I am here for you in your grief." Although the feelings and dynamics become more complicated and mature in adulthood, the fundamentals are still present: trust, warmth, acceptance, and a challenge to grow.

Your history with love lives on in the present, represented in blueprint form, coded in the neuronal wiring of your brain. The love you receive in childhood sets the stage for the love you will be drawn to in adulthood.[6]

LOVE PATTERNS

The poignancy and preciousness experienced as love and longing are the result of repeatedly activated neuronal pathways. Specific neurons, termed mirror neurons, light up in the frontal cortex of the brain not only when we engage in a particular behavior, but also when we observe others engaging in a behavior or exhibiting a particular emotional state. Learning, speaking, and observing the emotional pain of others activates mirror neurons.[7] Most importantly for our purposes, mirror neurons probably explain how we learn the patterns of love.

You have been taught how to love and what to expect in your relationships through experiencing and observing love in your immediate family. The brain has two kinds of memory: explicit and implicit. While explicit memory includes memories for facts or data you may consciously bring into your awareness and verbalize, implicit memory in the right hemisphere is a storehouse for all we know but cannot consciously state. Implicit memory does not lend itself to conscious recall. There are aspects of your personal history that you have no conscious memory of but that are still present in your brain's implicit memory system. "Implicit memory is the brain's sole learning component in the first years of life, when mother and child are bound together through their limbic connection."[8]

Implicit memory is at play when you have an overreaction that does not match the actual events in the environment, or if you just "have a feeling" about someone or something; this may suggest that an earlier learning experience was triggered.[9] Early caregiver behavior is stored in the child's implicit memory. For example, if parents exhibit indifference and avoidance, then children grow up unconsciously expecting to experience, on some level, the same from those they love in adulthood.

Although you may not consciously remember difficult love experiences, they are recorded in your brain's neuronal wiring and not only impact whom you choose to pursue as a love interest, but also the stability of your relationships in adulthood.

As described in chapter 6, when we repeat the same experience over time, the brain begins to make shortcuts to more quickly decipher the information. When you read a passage in a book, you may not notice a typographical error because the brain automatically fills in this data for you. Similarly, your brain expects to experience a specific pattern of love in relationships. Your brain essentially has a rough draft for how it expects love to proceed (if you expect others to be comforting and loving toward you or if you expect others to be guarded and emotionally unavailable to you) and creates shortcuts by filling in the dots to repeat this love scenario in your relationships. Even when a relationship experience is not exactly the same as your love history but has some similar details, it initially will be interpreted by the brain as the same as your past experience, and you will likely respond in the way you have in the past. As the authors of *A General Theory of Love* elaborate on these insights, "Because human beings remember with neurons, we are disposed to see more of what we have already seen, hear anew what we have heard most often, think just what we have always thought."[10]

In the dating world, it is common to hear others referring to "chemistry" and wanting to feel the "spark" with a potential new love. The experience of sparks or romantic chemistry is not consistently indicative of a relationship's health or capacity to provide lasting contentment. A hot crush is not the same as a mutually fulfilling and trusting connection and may reflect finding a match for your difficult love history. Recalling Hebb's theory from the last chapter, "cells that fire together wire together,"[11] a spark may simply mean that this particular romantic match is being lit by your previously existing wiring.

LOVE PATTERNS REPEAT

If early in life loving one or both of your caretakers left you feeling rejected, dismissed, or undervalued, then these are the feelings you will implicitly call up when you experience love in your adult relationships. "A child tunes in to the emotional patterns of parents and stores them. In later life, if he spots a close match, the key slides in the psychobiologic lock, the tumblers fall home, and he falls *in love*."[12]

You may not be conscious of why, but you may pick undependable, inattentive lovers who dismiss your emotional experiences. When you date someone who is kind and openly loving toward you, it may be hard to feel the spark because he does not match your early learning history and resulting neuronal wiring. You may not like this or consciously want it, but your brain is accustomed to relationships proceeding a certain way and, in the absence of new experience, will continually pull you toward that original model. "When one woman looks at an attractive man, she sees someone who wants to possess her and stifle her creativity; another sees a lonely soul who needs mothering and is crying out for her to do it; a third sees a playboy who must be seduced away from his desirable and unworthy mistress. Every one of them knows what she sees and never doubts the identity of the man in front of her faithful retinas, her fanciful brain."[13]

When something is familiar, whether it is a math problem or a relationship dynamic, it means your brain has learned that particular sequence quite well; the neuronal wiring is firmly in place, and the brain expends less energy doing the familiar than the unfamiliar. Many people report that, although they may not like a particular relationship dynamic that tends to repeat, the familiarity allows them to feel an odd sense of control because it is something they have managed all of their lives. It is often more frightening for people to imagine taking on a healthy relationship than to continue repeating a destructive relationship dynamic.

Love patterns also repeat because difficult childhood dynamics are typically tinged with intrigue. This intrigue in adulthood may create an exhilaration based on the fantasy that if the adult romantic relationship is a success, a painful past will be overcome. Difficult earlier dynamics may be repeated as a more successful and powerful adult sees an opportunity for a do-over. What was once a powerless little girl dependent on a distant or emotionally absent parent becomes a grown woman who finds an aloof and noncommittal man to be a sexy challenge.

An example of how the past may repeat is seen in the case of Diana. Diana felt unloved by her father, who was consistently preoccupied with his work and traveled for long stretches of time. As a young adult, Diana finds herself repeatedly drawn to men who are consumed by their work, periodically providing her with adoring attention followed by long periods of emotional distance. This is because what was a hurtful and disappointing relationship in childhood with her father was also the one set of circumstances in which Diana most wanted to feel special and cherished. Although Diana's father was not there for her in an emotional sense, every so often he would buy her something special or they would have a grand outing together. Like receiving a tiny slice of scrumptious cake, Diana was left longing for more. As an adult, Diana has only felt cherished and special in a relationship context where a highly desirable man with an ultraimportant schedule carves out small slivers of time for her.

In the process of therapy, Diana discovered what had been hidden—"Only men who are busy and aloof are worthy of my time." She felt that if she were able to win over this type of man, it would provide her with the sorely needed special love and acceptance she never received from her father.

Diana felt sexually charged by the mysterious and remote type who reproduced in her a sense of unfulfilled desire. These men lacked the emotional capacity to provide her with a stable, loving relationship, and so her needs for acceptance and consistent love continued to go unmet. Each time her romantic partner would avoid or ignore her, Diana felt the same rejection she felt by her father as a child, and she would become anxious and clingy. Eventually the relationship would destruct, and Diana would be left to feel all alone again, unworthy of love and vulnerable to repeating the same pattern.

It is important to understand the underpinnings of romantic love so as to recognize when you are engaging in a rigid pattern of loving that is self-defeating. Without new learning (new types of romantic partners who have the emotional capacity to be consistently loving toward you), these same patterns will continue to activate.

Neuronal plasticity is powerful. Our brains have the capacity to develop new patterns of circuitry and ways of being in the world through interactions with others. This may be achieved as long as you are willing to engage new types of men who are dissimilar to what you have experienced before. Even if your past experiences with love are inconsistent or unfulfilling, by engaging love in a new way and picking healthy romantic partners who have the capacity for care and emotional attunement, you will permanently alter your brain's love pattern.

RELATIONSHIPS SET THE STAGE

Christina grew up in a household where her parents, both professionals, were alcoholics. Christina's emotional needs went habitually and consistently unmet. Her father had a ferocious temper and, although not physically harmful, could be sharply critical and emotionally cruel. Every day in Christina's early childhood was a letdown. She would arrive home from school excited to share something about her day only to be met with angry, fighting, intoxicated parents. Christina adapted to this environment by sacrificing her needs and sense of self for the needs of her parents. She acted as perfectly pleasing as possible so as to feel more in control of her father's unpredictable eruptions and her mother's emotional withdrawal. Christina fixed potential problems on her own so that her parents would never have to be bothered, including difficulties in school, problems with friends, and even paying the electric bill on occasion. Over time, she no longer felt excited to share her accomplishments with her parents, let alone her difficulties. Instead, like a sponge, Christina absorbed the tension.

Christina attended so diligently to her family that she lost years of attending to her own life and missed forming a solid sense of self. A childhood spent overfunctioning for her parents left Christina as an adult with a wide swath of missing information about her identity. She came into treatment with little sense of herself. She could not articulate her likes and dislikes. Her professional goals were unformed. Her needs in intimate relationships were unexplored. While we worked to uncover and develop her sense of self, Christina's attention continually returned to pleasing others and being concerned with men finding her desirable.

It became apparent that Christina was unable to care for herself unless she was in a partnered relationship. She would only go to the grocery store or to the gym if she knew that her boyfriend might be coming by her apartment. She wanted to feel in shape for him and wanted to offer him food. When Christina's boyfriend was not present or when she was between relationships, she felt despair. When alone, Christina had little will to take care of her apartment, go to the gym, or eat healthfully. She would "hate on" her body and harshly criticize herself as being lazy and unmotivated. Christina's mood lifted only when a man came back into her life, and then she would put all of her attention into appearing physically desirable for him.

The partners Christina chose were men cast in the role of her father, men she could never please because they were uniformly self-consumed. When one of these men criticized her, Christina would spiral into her childhood pattern of striving to fix the problem while chastising herself as hopeless and unworthy of love. Occasionally, Christina's sense of self would briefly surface, and she would try to break up with a particular romantic partner. She was almost always drawn back into these destructive relationships. It was the only way Christina knew herself. When she was not living out this old storyline with a new romantic partner, Christina felt empty and estranged from herself.

Neurons respond to experience; the more you choose healthy romantic connections, the more your brain will grow to expect a different relationship drama to unfold in your life.[14] In order to gain control over dysfunctional love patterns, you must try out new love patterns.

Initially, new types of men may not bring the rush of adrenaline or instant validation to which you are accustomed. That is not to say that a spark will not develop with a man who is outside of your comfort zone, but it will take time for a new love pattern to be established. Engaging new types of romantic partners is similar to going to a foreign country for the first time; you may feel awkward, as you do not know how to speak the language or how to navigate the land, but you will leave feeling enriched and more hopeful about your future.

Relationships should feel like a secure base, not an emotional trigger for the psychic wounds of your childhood. If this is an unfamiliar feeling for you, then choose healthy partners despite yourself; do this again and again until you become accustomed to a healthy pattern. In Christina's case, it took effort and she had setbacks, but she is learning to push herself into different dating experiences. With this persistence, she is establishing a new love pattern.

TAKE STOCK OF YOUR CASTING DIRECTOR TENDENCIES

Take an inventory of your past and current relationship productions. As you become more fully aware of your love history and how your needs were met or unmet, you will develop a greater ability to see others as they really are. Ask yourself if you are playing the same role you did as a child. Have you adopted the role of one of your parents or even the role you played in a previous romantic relationship? Become fully cognizant of whom you are choosing to become romantic with and assess whether that person reminds you of a dysfunctional relationship from your past.

A faulty love pattern is seen in the case of Susan. Susan grew up in an emotionally neglectful household, and her parents contentiously divorced when she was eight. The divorce emotionally fractured Susan. Her father was a safe spot in her life, and she was no longer able to see him frequently. Susan's mother was often so preoccupied with getting her own needs met that when Susan expressed sadness or anger about the divorce, her mother would respond with how difficult the divorce was on *her*, thus never validating Susan's emotional experience. At times when Susan would express upset, her mother would shame her—"Why are you upset? I am the one that has to work two jobs now to take care of you and your sister by myself!" Through the years, Susan thwarted her needs and unconsciously began to take care of her mother. She would ask about her mother's day and her feelings, likes, and dislikes and received little of this emotional care in return. Now, as an adult, Susan finds herself repeating a pattern. Initially she feels intense chemistry and closeness with her partners, but as time passes, she begins to feel a building sense of resentment.

When romantic partners express a benign request, such as a desire to attend a baseball game or to change plans, suddenly, out of nowhere, Susan becomes enraged with her partner. Although Susan's needs were inconsistently met in childhood, she reversed this theme as an adult into "I will get my needs met no matter what the cost." The anger she experiences with her romantic partners helps Susan to feel in control, thus keeping her from feeling the vulnerability she experienced as a child. She unintentionally creates relationships that are similar to her childhood in that they are filled with anger and a general lack of empathy.

As Susan became more in touch with the grief and emotional neglect she experienced as a child, she was better able to find a balance with her romantic partners and form a committed relationship. Rather than becoming angry over inconsequential events, Susan learned to speak more openly about her fears and past hurt. When Susan chose partners who could respond to her past with empathy, she felt attended to for the first time in her life and no longer became angry and controlling when they expressed a difference of opinion.

Take an inventory of your relationship history and how you may cast romantic partners according to your background. Reflect on the ways in which attending to your needs and the needs of your partners may be out of balance and work on identifying where you first learned the love patterns that are causing problems today.

Consider the following questions: Did you feel you could rely on your caretakers for most of what you needed? Consider whether you were overly gratified and given what you wished without question. How do you repeat past relationship dynamics with caregivers in your current relationships with men? Are the men you choose similar to your mother or your father in healthy ways or unhealthy ways? Do you tend to repeatedly deny your needs in your relationships? Do you sell yourself out by telling yourself, "I don't want to ask for what I want because I will appear dramatic and needy"? Or perhaps you have an explosive approach; is it your way or the highway? Do you get your needs met on the sly, secretly, thus never having to fully depend on or be open with your partners? This is seen in people who have affairs, addictions, and secret lives separate from their significant others. Are you in a relationship without closeness or intimate communication? How is this similar to your early relationships with your caretakers? Do you give little room for your significant other to have autonomy and a life separate from you? Are you so entirely absorbed by your partner's needs that, in a way, there is no "you" separate from your partner? Individuals who answer "yes" to some of these questions may lack sufficient self-awareness and use relationships as a way to fabricate an identity.

Recognize that you will continue to suffer until you become fully aware of how you replay a self-defeating script in your adult romantic relationships. Below are a few common relationship dynamics that signal the repetition of a problem love pattern from your past. See if you recognize yourself in one or more of these categories. Once you identify the theme you are repeating in your romantic relationships, you will be better equipped to develop more fulfilling love patterns.

INSTANT FIREWORKS

How many times have you watched a scene in a movie where a chance encounter between two attractive characters yields love at first sight? Although it is important in romantic love to have chemistry, initially seeing stars is often a sign that the man involved may trigger a relationship dynamic from your past.

Instant fireworks often occur for women who camouflage their issues with a new man. Instead of working through a difficult attachment history or negative self-image, they may place their partners on a pedestal and forgo developing themselves. Placing romantic partners on a pedestal is a way to make up for a self-worth deficit. By failing to harness your own self-esteem, you live off of his. If he is confident, sexy, and high achieving, then suddenly you feel better about yourself, almost as if he is you. As a general rule of thumb, the higher your expectations for perfection from your partner, the more depleted and inadequate you may feel about yourself.

Judgment is impaired by having expectations for romantic perfection. If you are lost in the dreamy clouds of assuring yourself that you have found a perfect ten, it becomes impossible to make an accurate assessment of who the person really is. If you idealize your partners or place them on a pedestal, you are lost in an illusion of perfection that is destined to dissolve.[15] When the façade cracks, you are left to feel disappointed and shocked at the reality of who sits before you.

Attaching your self-esteem to an idealized other is often related to childhood dynamics of a parent who would pop in with fun and pop out leaving sadness and disappointment. Children who grow up with a parent who is inconsistently available become accustomed to subsisting on the good times and accepting despair in the disappointing times.

Ask yourself if you are prone to idealizing your partners or making an accurate assessment of who your partners really are. Do you have difficulty with the getting-to-know-you process that dating involves and, as a result, sacrifice learning who your partners are in favor of instant chemistry? Reflect on what it is that you consider unlovable or wrong about yourself. Is it something you work to camouflage by being associated with a highly desirable man? If that is the case, remind yourself that no matter where you go or whom you date, you will not escape how you feel about yourself.

THE FIXER UPPER

In contrast to instant fireworks, the fixer upper comes when you recognize your potential partner's imperfections but take on the project of making him over to become what it is you desire. Like instant fireworks, the fixer upper is a way to manage a depleted and inadequate sense of self. Without working to fulfill yourself, you place all of your energy into getting him to step up and become the man you believe he should be.

You never have to acknowledge your unresolved issues and depleted sense of self if you put all of your emotional energy into getting your partner to see his flaws and work on improving himself. This dynamic is seen in women who frequently make heartfelt complaints about their partners, including, "Why can't he call and let me know where he is? . . . He needs to work on communicating better . . . He has to step up to the plate . . . He truly needs therapy . . . Men really are from Mars." Women who chronically engage the fixer upper hold a firmly rooted belief that if they work really hard, they can transform their sextimacy partner into Prince Charming.

Research shows that if a relationship starts off poorly, it is unlikely to improve. People who believe their relationships will improve over time with greater commitment or even marriage often end up divorced.[16] Early differences in a relationship, including unresolved conflict, lack of mutual affection, and impaired reciprocal communication, do not typically improve in time or with hard work and, in fact, typically never improve. If you are constantly trying to get your partner to step it up by encouraging him to take on a goal or challenge or to become more committed to you, it is unlikely that he is ever going to do so in the context of your relationship. People rarely change unless it is on their terms.

The fixer upper is often related to a childhood love pattern of wishing and hoping a parent will change and working tirelessly to get a parent to do the right thing—all to no avail. The reality is people evolve in the direction they wish to evolve. We cannot control the paths of others.

Do you often lament, "This guy just doesn't get it," or "He acts like a Neanderthal," and yet you continue to pursue the same types who need your help? How do you explain to yourself, let alone to others, that all you want is a guy who knows what he wants and is ready for commitment even though you choose to consistently date men who obviously do not have the emotional maturity for meaningful commitment? This is equivalent to wanting to be a physician but enrolling in cooking school—you are not providing yourself with the basic necessities for creating the emotional intimacy and relationship fulfillment you seek.

If you continue to date fixer uppers, your actions are inconsistent with a true desire for emotional intimacy and suggest that you need to focus your attention spotlight not on others but on yourself.

BREAKING UP AND MAKING UP

Breaking up and making up reflects an obsessive pattern of alternating between idealizing and devaluing a love interest. Each time your partner makes you feel good and secure, you make up, and the good times roll. When you experience your partner as uncaring, disappointing, or unappreciative, you break up and your self-esteem plummets. With each successive reiteration of the idealizing/devaluing pattern, the good times are shorter, and the bad times are longer. The pattern lives on because neither partner wants to engage in the process of acknowledging the toxic nature of the relationship, grieving what it cannot be, and moving on.

Sextimacy often reflects a breakup/makeup pattern; each time the romance dwindles, the woman tells herself, "Never again," only to find herself making up the next time her sextimacy partner turns on the charm. Women who repeat the breakup/makeup pattern often do so because they alternate between becoming angry at the lack of care and love they are receiving to feeling rapture when their partner makes even the smallest gesture of care.

Women who repeatedly make up with their partners tend to hate on themselves for what they believe they did wrong in the relationship. As opposed to considering their partner's lack of capacity for commitment and emotional intimacy, these women focus on how their appearance or behavior led to the deterioration of the relationship. Then they work frantically to redeem themselves through winning back the one who keeps disappointing.

Women who are caught in this pattern often have a history of loss or emotional trauma, which they have not effectively processed or grieved. They may blame themselves for the earlier pain. Each time the woman in this hopeless love pattern fails to end the relationship and chooses to make up, she is giving herself a reprieve from the unresolved earlier loss and sadness.

Recognize how much your self-esteem depends on the status of your breakup/makeup relationship. Consider whether you are avoiding feeling sadness or grief from your past by not ending a toxic relationship. Remind yourself that, as hard as it is to end important relationships, the person you leave is still alive and existing in the universe, and your show must go on. Find ways to manage these feelings without sacrificing your self-esteem. Reread chapters 4 and 6 in this book and develop outlets for healthy coping.

CATCHIN' FEELINGS

You may tell yourself that you are in a particular relationship for the sex alone and then before you know it, attachment hormones start doing their work. You may not wish it, but poof, suddenly you have become emotionally attached to someone who has no interest in knowing you. Once attached, you are "catchin' feelings," and you become self-critical when the man is inattentive and dismissive. It would be best to recognize that you picked a partner who is incapable of providing you with real emotional intimacy, but more likely you turn on yourself and wonder what is wrong with you that he does not seek you out more or make any effort to get to know you on an intimate level.

A catchin' feelings scenario is characterized by intermittent, exciting hookups followed by periods of your partner's withdrawal and absence. Women who are caught in this dynamic often feel they are constantly settling for romantic leftovers. There is no real care involved in this, but women who settle for it are uncomfortable with partners who consistently want to care for and know them.

Make no mistake: Casual sex is anything but easy and casual. It takes a considerable amount of self-deception to be sexually involved with someone who has little interest in knowing the real you. Consider whether you engage in self-deception by telling yourself and others that you are only in a particular relationship for the sex, or you are only looking for fun with your romantic partners with no commitment.

Are you being entirely honest with yourself? Do you have any desire to know and be known by your romantic partners? If so, recognize that you are settling for a self-defeating love pattern that will, likely, never deliver real intimacy or care. Perhaps you have felt emotionally neglected for most of your life. If that is the case, notice how you are now choosing partners whose treatment of you extends that neglect.

If you often fall into a catchin' feelings love pattern, you can defeat this pattern by putting greater energy into the other interests in your life. Stop settling for the scraps in romantic relationships. Develop healthy male friendships without the early introduction of sex.

I WOULD RATHER BE UNKNOWN THAN DISLIKED

If you are repeating the unknown/known dynamic, then you have a tendency to choose men who find you wonderfully desirable, as long as they do not have to deal with anything as messy or complicated as your emotional needs. Your job in this type of relationship is to keep it all pretty on the outside because your partner suddenly becomes inattentive and uninterested when you express a need or negative emotion. For women in the unknown/known love pattern, ensuring they are liked trumps everything, and they are willing to morph themselves into whatever is necessary to hold their love's interest. They tend to believe the price of a good relationship is appearing hot at all times and perfectly pleasing. They are unaccustomed to back-and-forth interactions, where all topics are open for discussion and acceptance permeates.

The unknown/known love pattern often occurs for women who as children were treated wonderfully when they were pleasing and were punished when they were anything less. Women in this pattern tend to believe that their negative feelings are shameful and need to be hidden. They perpetually engage partners who only want to see their rosy side. They are so familiar with being dismissed or ignored when they express anything negative that they have learned never to show their emotional side. These women tend to pick men who are comfortable with nothing more complicated than a perfect little doll.

Do you pick partners who do not want to get to know the whole woman? It is important to broaden your spectrum to connecting with your worth on more dimensions than merely being liked. If you cannot learn to tolerate others' dislike or rejection, it will be close to impossible to find a loving relationship.

In order to be you, imperfections and all, you need to show your entire self to those you care for most. Work toward becoming at ease talking with others about what distresses you and about your emotional world. The more you practice, the more comfortable you will become in sharing your whole self.

TRY OUT NEW RELATIONSHIP DYNAMICS

You can alter your love map on a neuronal level by loving healthy people. When you engage in a new relationship, you create a new, shared reality, and healthy or unhealthy, this new reality shapes your identity. Experiencing a difficult history with love but pairing with someone who has a healthy love map will ease old emotional wounds. Each time you mutually exchange care and interest, a new experience of love is incorporated into the way your brain is wired.

It takes courage to forge a relationship with someone who desires to know you and is capable of reciprocating your care for him. This kind of attachment may feel unfamiliar and uncomfortable. Yet, it could change long-held, core assumptions and help you to begin knowing yourself in a positive new way.

As explored previously, your implicit memory uses shortcuts to get around the hard work of learning new information. These shortcuts will tell you that relationships generally proceed in the manner you experienced them in the past. Allow yourself to become open to a new storyline. Try to rewrite the script so your relationships proceed in the direction you desire, and lose your preconceived dedication to a particular type of male personality.

Relate and connect in ways that are not romantic. Consider psychotherapy, where you will have the new experience of feeling understood by someone who genuinely wants to know you so that you may better know yourself.

KISS A FROG

In Dweck's theory of success, she found that the mindset you hold about your abilities (fixed or growth) impacts how successful you may be in developing productive relationships. In one study, people were asked to describe a time in their lives when they were painfully rejected by a significant other. The stories people told were all sad and even heartbreaking, but mindset determined how effectively people managed their particular situation.

Those who held a fixed mindset about themselves tended to feel damaged as a result of the rejection, as if an ultimate judgment of being unlovable was cast on them. Because this judgment is experienced by fixed-mindset individuals as permanent and irreparable, they have no strategies for managing these awful feelings. Instead of working through these emotions, fixed-mindset individuals tend to put their attention into exacting revenge or getting back at the one who wounded them. When growth-mindset individuals experienced hurt and sadness, they considered ways in which they would proceed differently in their next relationship. Growth-mindset individuals focused on forgiveness, letting go, and improving specific relationship skills in the future.[17]

In a separate study of college students, researchers categorized students according to their views of relationships. A fixed view of relationships means you believe relationships are either meant to be or not meant to be, while a growth view means you believe healthy relationships take time and effort to develop. Findings indicate that students who hold strong growth beliefs endorse having longer-term relationships and fewer one-night stands, while those students who hold fixed beliefs tend to end relationships at the first sign of discontent.[18]

If you see your entire worth as dependent on your relationships and believe relationships are either meant to be or not, then you look for men who do not challenge you to grow. Sextimacy is the same experience again and again—a series of brief liaisons that provide temporary self-validation but do not give you the opportunity to improve your communication skills or develop more emotional self-awareness. As soon as you no longer feel wanted by a sextimacy partner, you move on to the fresh excitement of another temporary liaison.

Holding a mindset that relationships are either meant to be or not meant to be leads to a fantasy that, on a very special day in the future, you will find your Prince Charming and all will be right in the world. The reality is you need to take the time not just to kiss a number of frogs, but also to get to know your partners. This is the path for making better choices.

Approach each date or romantic experience with the mindset that eventually you will meet the right person. What is far more difficult than marriage or finding a boyfriend is discovering a match that is fulfilling for the long term, a match in which you mutually attend to one another's needs. Adopting an outlook that dating is a learning process that *eventually* will result in a long-term relationship will enable you to maintain your self-esteem and more fully appreciate the experience.

LEARN TO BEAR REJECTION

Rejecting undesirable mates represents a normal drive to partner with a suitable match. At the same time, the drive to avoid rejection, at any cost, is strong for most. Rejection is difficult, and when you encounter it, the brain reminds you of other times in your life when you felt unwanted.

Rejection may occur in a relatively benign or an extremely hurtful context, but almost everyone has experienced feeling unwanted. Were you the last picked for your team in physical education class? Did your parents dismiss you when you were upset or angry? Did you feel disliked by a peer or excluded? Were you abandoned emotionally or physically by caretakers? All of these experiences, big or small, burn a place on the human heart, a place of vulnerability that is often accompanied by a personal conviction that you will never, under any circumstances, allow yourself to feel rejection again.

There is a direct relationship between how unwanted and cast-off one felt in childhood and how much one engages in self-protection in adulthood. Some have an ability to shrug off rejection. For others it is more difficult. The more you can learn to tolerate rejection, without a loss to your self-esteem, the better equipped you will be to know where you stand in your relationships and to deepen the emotional intimacy.

Jennifer's story offers an illustration of how self-destructive the fear of rejection can be. Jennifer, a thirty-five-year-old high-achieving professional, struggled with lifelong depression. Through psychotherapy treatment, Jennifer's depressive symptoms improved considerably, and she began to notice all that she had missed in life. She was divorced and recognized that she had married someone with whom she had little in common and who rebuffed emotional intimacy. Because Jennifer wanted to avoid herself emotionally, this love pattern worked for her at that time. As she improved, Jennifer's sense of self and a desire for closeness evolved. She began to date a man who not only shared her love for music and studying Buddhism, but who was also interested in her emotional world. She enjoyed this new kind of attachment to a man, and for the first time in her life, felt known by another human being in more than a superficial way.

However, at one point in their relationship, Jennifer's new love began to pull back. Eventually, Jennifer's partner communicated that he was unsure of her feelings for him, and this was causing him to retreat. Although Jennifer knew how strongly she felt for him, she could not directly put her feelings on the table. I asked her, "Why not let him know how important this relationship is to you and that you are over the moon with delight?" She responded, "Well there is always the possibility he won't feel the same way." So Jennifer chose to say nothing, and the relationship faded away.

Communicating about how you feel in a particular relationship may allow for the intimacy in the relationship to grow, or it may inform you that the man is incapable of providing what you desire. Although you may be rejected, which is to say he does not share your feelings, you *need* to know this information in order to move forward with your long-term best interest in mind.

Relationships and even marriages have the potential to last for years with chronic discontent. The unhappiness often goes unspoken because one or both partners are paralyzed by the belief that speaking about their areas of conflict will cause the other person to leave. So the relationship endures, and yes, rejection is not directly felt, but the cost is great—years of dissatisfaction traded so as never to risk feeling unwanted or rejected.

Without the ability to tolerate the possibility of experiencing rejection, you may unknowingly sabotage your relationships. Low self-esteem and fear of abandonment can lead to an overanxious energy in a relationship where you are ever vigilant for criticism or distance. Questions such as, "Did you go out last night? . . . Who were you with? . . . Who were you talking to? . . . Can I check your phone/text log?" convey your expectation that eventually your partner will no longer want you in his life. Although this is a way of protecting yourself from the pain of rejection, ultimately this type of vigilance erodes feelings of closeness and mutual acceptance.

Instead of anxious vigilance, remind yourself that all the checking, guessing, and questioning in the world will not make it any easier to deal with relationship loss and may contribute to its occurrence. Notice whether you tend not to express your needs and feelings in your romantic relationships out of fear your partner will bolt. Committing yourself to a random hookup pattern or worse, a lifetime with someone who is not rising to what you want, sacrifices your happiness and potential. Learn to endure short-term, albeit intensely negative, feelings of rejection in order to get a life and partner that will fulfill you.

When someone you are attached to becomes remote and you feel unwanted by them, a natural longing and desire to seek proximity follows. The longer you are connected or attached to someone, the more that attachment is wired in your brain. Allow time for the loss to metabolize and move through your system. Remind yourself that no one is wanted at all times by everyone in their lives; it is simply impossible. You cannot live your life fully and openly without feeling unwanted from time to time.

Redirect your attention spotlight on areas in your life where you do feel wanted and needed. Pick yourself up and affiliate, build new relationships, and connect with volunteer groups or your work projects.

DWELL IN THE DARK

Occasionally dwelling in negative thoughts or feelings about people with whom you are close is a normal part of the human experience. Acknowledging what you like about others and what is harder for you to tolerate provides needed self-awareness so that, if for no other reason, you will not be blindsided by the sudden realization of who really stands before you. The difficulty arises if you shame yourself for having such thoughts or mindlessly deny the nature of the experience you are having with another.

Women who use relationships as their only avenue for self-validation tend to rationalize the bad behavior of others to avoid conflict. If you do not allow yourself to acknowledge what may be unsound about your romantic partner's character, then you are missing important data that will tell you whether the relationship will ultimately serve you equitably.

All thoughts, good and bad, about the people in your life may reflect something about the person's capacity to give. Sextimacy, for many women, means giving up assessing how their partners make them feel. Perhaps you have noticed something about one of your partners that you do not like or a need you have that is not being addressed but ignore it to avoid conflict. If you deny the existence of your needs, making an accurate assessment as to whether or not a particular relationship will ultimately satisfy you is impossible. Once you begin to acknowledge your needs in the present moment, you will be free to acknowledge to yourself and to your partner if those needs are not being met.

For example, Samantha finally scored the guy of her dreams—good job, attractive, successful, the life of the party. The two worked together for a little more than a year when he finally asked her out. Samantha was thrilled to be liked by someone who seemed to have it all and instantly felt a surge in her self-esteem. At first the dating went well, but in time Samantha's mood changed. In our sessions, Samantha would relate the details of their encounters, all of which sounded lovely: making dinner together, going out to exciting events, spending time with good friends. However, she seemed sad as she recalled these happy times. When I asked about this, she said, "I wish he would ask more about me. I feel I know him, but he knows very little about who I am, other than what I like to do." As quickly as she uttered these thoughts, she took them away. "He has so much going on; his job is stressful, so it helps him to talk about his work, and it makes me feel good to be there for him . . . once his job calms down, I am sure he will want to hear more about me."

Samantha knew something meaningful about her new love interest. He had difficulty taking in another's perspective and was fairly self-absorbed. She was unwilling to dwell on these darker thoughts or fully acknowledge the negative aspects of this man. She pushed these considerations away in favor of maintaining the relationship. By not attending to what was missing in their relationship, Samantha enabled his bad behavior to continue and essentially endorsed his failure to know her more deeply.

Dark data do not have to mean the end of a relationship; whatever you notice can be discussed between you and your partner, so you may accurately assess whether the relationship has the potential to grow. If your partner refuses to participate in this discussion, you have learned that there is little likelihood of ever having a mutually satisfying bond with him.

In another case, Jenna grew up with a physically impaired single mother who had severe multiple sclerosis and was unable to do simple tasks. Jenna was her gofer, assistant, nurse, and mother. In her early twenties, Jenna met Joe, who was studying to become a physical therapist. As the two began to talk more intimately, they discovered they shared similar backgrounds. Joe grew up in a household where his mother suffered panic attacks so intense that she was often unable to leave the family home. Joe's father absorbed himself in his work and was rarely around the family. Jenna was intimately familiar with Joe's suffering, as she experienced a similar burden of responsibility in childhood. Through openly talking about their backgrounds, Jenna and Joe helped one another with their weaknesses and found ways to communicate when either felt taken advantage of by the other. The shared empathy and compassion they felt for one another enabled Jenna and Joe to forge a new kind of relationship, one that neither had experienced in the past.

In order to see others clearly—that is, as they really are—you must let your ongoing experience of your partners fully register without a loss of self-esteem. Allow yourself to dwell on your darker concerns about your romantic partners—without engaging in self-deception or criticizing yourself as dramatic or overly emotional. Simply allow yourself to consider all aspects of the person in front of you.

CONCLUSION

Just like anything, in order to grow you need a goal and a plan for how to get there. If you are reading this book, chances are you want an emotionally and sexually satisfying relationship where you know your partner and feel known and cared for in return. Now tell yourself that all of this will happen as long as you are willing to work on growing as an individual, challenging yourself with new types of relationships, and attending to how you experience your partners. Commit to your goal of a successful relationship through resisting sextimacy encounters and being direct with men about what it is you seek. As you work on developing your relationship proficiency, find outlets for fulfillment separate from men and ways to become comfortable being alone (see chapter 6).

If you build a satisfying life filled with meaning and purpose, love will follow. When you do find the right man, he will be the cherry on the ice cream sundae of your life, but just the cherry.

8

GOOD GIRLS

Developing an Authentic Sexual Self

Eliza was a good girl. Growing up, she lived for straight A's on her report card and seeing the pride in her parents' eyes. It seemed everything Eliza touched turned to gold; she achieved academically, excelled athletically, and easily developed relationships with others. Her peers and relatives gently teased her for always being so good. "Here comes Miss Perfect," they would say. Eliza was more surprised than anyone when, toward the end of high school, she began to hook up with classmates on a regular basis. After each sextimacy event, she felt shame and guilt because deep down she believed that only "bad girls" hooked up. Eliza ceaselessly self-criticized and berated herself for engaging in these sexual experiences.

Nevertheless, when someone attractive desired her, Eliza felt a rush of excitement that invariably culminated in sex. She kept these sextimacy events and her self-contempt a secret and comported herself as being sexually innocent. Through the years, Eliza had difficulty sticking with committed relationships because they did not produce the rush of instant validation and the high of feeling desirable. Following the typical sextimacy pattern, she worked to please her partners—enjoying sex solely through their enjoyment of her. By the time Eliza came to therapy, she had been married for five years, she was unfulfilled sexually, and she was considering having an affair.

THE MAKINGS OF A GOOD GIRL

An omnipresent image in our culture is a woman effortlessly accomplishing multiple tasks—work, school, sports, friendship, romance, caregiving, and parenting—all the while appearing sexually attractive. It is an image that women often feel compelled to approximate. For many girls, the more they perceive others valuing them, the more they experience themselves as lovable and worthwhile. By the time girls turn into women, they may have become quite accustomed to others not taking their feelings seriously or wanting to know them on an emotionally intimate level. These women often turn to external avenues for self-validation, picking partners and products that take them further away from self-knowledge and emotional intimacy.

Cultural and family messages about appearing good and perfect leave women vulnerable to the idea that fixing the external will bring a wealth of contentment, including a spicy sex life. This premise may be pursued in many different ways—liposuction, breast augmentation, lip augmentation, Botox, dressing seductively. There are even specific products designed to spruce up women's genitalia, including dressing up pubic hair with a Brazilian wax and doctoring vaginal "odor" with perfumes.

Little exists in popular culture about how sex can be pleasurable for women, how young women may enjoy their first sexual experience, or how women may better understand their sexuality separate from simply pleasing men. One of the consequences of this hyper-focus on the external is that it leads many women toward a disconnected and unfulfilling sex life. They may complain that sex has become compartmentalized as something else on the to-do list—a task to check off, while the experience itself is empty and unfulfilling.

Family and culture offer young women very little guidance in terms of female anatomy and sexual fulfillment or permission to fully understand their own sexuality. Because the ways in which women respond sexually are less overt and more complicated than men's, women who do not have basic knowledge of their sexual anatomy and permission to explore have difficulty understanding their sexuality and enjoying their sexual experiences. Beginning in adolescence, many girls only hear from authority figures about the dangers of STDs and pregnancy, or how guys are "out for one thing" and how it is important not to "get a reputation."

Early in their development, girls are warned about sex and conditioned to become more fearful than curious. In lieu of understanding her sexual self, a kind of anxiety invades the young woman's burgeoning sexuality. This anxiety even permeates interactions with other women. Young women often do not talk with one another in meaningful ways about how they are discovering their desire and pleasure. When they do talk, what they say is full of contradictions reflecting the anxiety and conflict they experience. They may talk in terms of wanting to keep their "numbers low," debriefing after a hookup experience or consoling one another during a pregnancy scare.

In spite of adult tactics, many adolescents remain sexually active. The Centers for Disease Control and Prevention (CDC) reports that 46 percent of high school students say they have had sexual intercourse.[1] The rate for boys and girls is about the same. Fourteen percent had sex with four or more partners. More telling in terms of current sexual activity, CDC data show 53.1 percent of twelfth-grade females reporting that they have experienced intercourse with at least one person during the previous three months.[2] A Guttmacher Institute report covering a slightly wider age span reports, "By the time they reach 19, seven in 10 never-married teens have engaged in sexual intercourse."[3]

Whatever the precise number, many adolescent girls are engaging in sex, and they are doing so with a tremendous amount of anxiety, a lack of knowledge about female sexual response patterns, and a lack of pleasure, conditions that set the stage for a good-girl-bad-girl dichotomy. It is when girls are in the dark about female sexuality and given little guidance or permission to understand themselves sexually (separate from pleasing men) that many young women waffle back and forth between sexual repression and promiscuity. Girls and women who are caught in this dichotomy swing between two poles: chaste enough to be perceived as a good girl while simultaneously addicted to the rush of feeling sexually desired.[4]

When I ask these young women about their sexual experiences, time and time again, I hear that they enjoyed making out or kissing but that the sex was unremarkable—"It was so-so," "Not the best," or "Fine." They do not bemoan this because for some women, the thrill of feeling sexually desired trumps orgasm.

Once the sextimacy event is over, they often feel guilty and swing back to the chaste good-girl persona. When another attractive guy comes around, the exhilaration of his desire makes the bad girl reappear. Swinging between these poles causes an inordinate amount of anxiety and tension for those who experience it and, perhaps even more importantly, keeps them in the dark about how they might get more from their romantic experiences.

A WAY OUT: SEXTIMACY

Sextimacy has women experiencing men's desire while remaining out of touch with their sexuality. Within a sextimacy encounter, the woman can convince herself that she appears both innocent and sexy. She might say, "I do not even know you," or "I don't usually do this." Sextimacy occurring as an isolated event can more easily be dismissed the next day. The women involved typically tell themselves they have no plans for another sextimacy event and rationalize that it occurred because they were intoxicated or swept away. Sextimacy becomes a way to compartmentalize sex from the rest of a woman's experience of herself.

For many women and young women in particular, the sexual conquest itself is neither sexually satisfying nor emotionally intimate. These women are not only disposed to disconnect from their bodies during the sexual encounter, but they also feel unconnected to their partners. This disconnection is entirely contrary to developing a healthy self-image or a pleasurable sexual life.

Each sextimacy event makes it more challenging for the woman to learn on her own how to enjoy sex with a monogamous partner. In effect, these experiences condition her to be disconnected from her own sexual response patterns, desires, and needs. It becomes difficult for her to make informed choices about sex in which her long-term best interest is the first priority.

Nonetheless, women typically report that they hope their hookups will one day turn into committed relationships, and they often initiate conversations with their partners about "taking it to the next level" or work in other ways to deepen the connection. Men, on the other hand, do not typically expect a hookup to turn into a romantic relationship. Sextimacy unilaterally meets the needs of men more than the needs of women. Some women are willing to accept this because they wish to feel desirable to men, and they have had little opportunity to understand their own interpersonal potential.

OBJECT OF DESIRE

Typically, sexual pleasure is addressed in popular culture from the male's perspective of a female being the object of his desire. Girls and women are frequently left with massive gaps in their understanding of sexual partnership from their own perspective. As discussed in chapter 2, the popularly described male gauge of considerations becomes for many women their gauge for what constitutes female attractiveness. They imagine what will be a turn-on or a turn-off for a male and then work to approximate that male ideal.

This external focus leaves some women uninformed about what drives their sexuality. With so few healthy models of female sexuality in the culture, many women believe they are not really supposed to enjoy sex or to see it from their own perspective because that would not conform to the good-girl ideal they have absorbed.

Most young women have very little space in which they may experience their sexuality in a safe manner that allows them to experiment and explore who they are as sexual beings. Some women come to appreciate sex solely through feeling wanted and desired by their partners and by seeing themselves through their partners' eyes. Developing an understanding for what drives their sexuality is not only essential for sexual fulfillment, but also for sex to be safe and fully consensual.

Forty-one percent of girls between the ages of fourteen and seventeen seen in urban health clinics report that they agreed to sex despite knowing they did not actually desire sex. Girls who consent to unwanted sex also report less condom use, which, of course, places them at increased risk for STDs and pregnancy.[5] Girls typically consent to sex without actually desiring it because of low self-esteem and to appease their partners. Similarly, as adults, many women report that their first sexual experience "just happened" or occurred in a way where they gave outward consent but internally remained disengaged. By agreeing to unwanted sex, girls maintain the positive vibes flowing in their relationships and attain a momentary sense of self-validation.

When women do not consent to sex for their own desired pleasure, they become vulnerable to risky, unfulfilling, or even nonconsensual sexual experiences.[6] Women disconnected from their sexual desire may be at a loss for knowing whether they want to have sex or are doing so only in order to feel the rush of a romantic partner's desire. Women who become addicted to the high of feeling wanted are vulnerable to impulsive sex.

INCREASE YOUR FITNESS FOR FULFILLING SEX

Although women have given birth to the entire human race, many still feel a sense of shame about what is "down there." The language used to describe female anatomy in popular culture today reinforces this shame, as it is often derogatory and leaves many women feeling guarded and unentitled to sexual pleasure. For instance, in *The Story of V*, Catherine Blackledge connects the term *cunt* to the originating benign words *cuneus* or *cleft*. Because a cleft or wedge is essentially the first thing an observer sees when looking at female anatomy, Blackledge theorizes that the term *cleft* was used in ancient times to refer to female genitalia: "What is visible is a pubic triangle, with a line running down the middle."[7] Further evidence for the connection between *cunt* and *cleft* is seen in cuneiform, ancient pictorial writing dating as early as 3500 BC, where the symbol for woman is "the image of cunt—a downwards-facing triangle with a line cleft down its middle."[8] This vulgar expression and others like it are taken personally today by women because of the contemptuous and disrespectful meaning with which they are now associated.

While women may have access to birth control and an array of options to express themselves sexually, the internalized sense of shame that some harbor disconnects them from their own sexual voice separate from striving to approximate an ideal standard of beauty that will attract male desire. The next section of this chapter is geared to helping you commit to no longer having sex without pleasure and desire and to developing your sexuality independent of pleasing men. Through exploring your sexual anatomy and response patterns, becoming aware of the beliefs you hold that stifle your sexual fulfillment, developing an ability to connect with pleasure in your life, and writing a new sexual storyline for yourself that includes *your* pleasure, you will learn to non-judgmentally accept your sexual self.

BECOMING COMFORTABLE IN YOUR OWN SKIN

There is an irony present in the tendency to sexualize girls and women so that they are treated by men and by themselves as sex objects, while at the same time, many girls and women possess no real understanding for their sexual preferences or knowledge of their sexual anatomy. There are many roadblocks to this understanding. The words *vagina* and *vulva* make people uncomfortable, so much so that many adults teach their children euphemisms that only reinforce the mystification of the vagina. Terms like *hoo-hoo*, *coochie*, *kitty*, *twat*, *cha-cha*, and of course the ever so clear *down there*, easily roll off the tongue for well-meaning parents and caregivers. The problem is not the terms themselves but using this type of language to the exclusion of meaningful discussion in which the child may develop a more nuanced understanding of her body and freely ask questions.

Many girls grow up to become women who believe that, because their anatomy and sexual response patterns are so mysterious and different from men's, it is a losing battle to try to gain sexual pleasure. Research indicates that the total prevalence of sexual dysfunction for women, including lack of interest in sex, inability to achieve orgasm, or experiencing pain during intercourse, is 43 percent.[9] In particular, younger women who are single and experience greater sexual instability in terms of partners and sexual activity feel increased stress around the sex act itself, which makes it more likely that they will experience sexual pain and anxiety. A recent large-scale study examining subjective sexual wellbeing across cultures demonstrated that women report less sexual satisfaction than men.[10] And many studies show that 10 percent of women have never experienced an orgasm, either with a partner or during masturbation.

With little direct communication and labeling, even by educated and feministic women, it is easy for girls to develop an internalized sense of shame and confusion about their own anatomy. Deep within the recesses of many women's minds is the thought that it is somehow unseemly or bad to physically explore their sexual anatomy. The lack of direct labeling about female anatomy contributes to the vulva region existing as a paradoxical no-man's-land for the woman and, yet, a place where men are permitted entrance. Knowing and accepting your body, your sexual anatomy, and how the two operate together is essential for a fulfilling sex life.

Adopt a mindset of acceptance for your body and calm curiosity about how it works. Embrace self-exploration. Read about female sexuality. Communicate with other women about female sexual response patterns. If you allow your sexual self to remain unexplored, confusion and mystery will impede your enjoyment of sex.

As you increase your fitness for enjoyable sex, notice whether your thoughts serve to block this exploration. For some women, feelings of embarrassment and shame surface when they attempt to explore. These feelings merely reflect the ways in which our world conditions many women to feel uncomfortable about their sexuality. Recognize that everything that occurs in your vulva is natural and is designed to support your enjoyment of sex.

For example, when pressed on this subject, some women tell me they feel ashamed of the smell and tart taste of the vagina and do not embrace pleasure out of fear that their vagina is unbecoming. In fact, as Blackledge outlines, maintaining vaginal pH is a way that the vagina remains healthy: "In the healthy premenopausal woman, vaginal pH should remain low, hovering around pH 4.0. That is, it's best to be acidic, or tart, but not as tart as a lemon (pH 2.0). More like a glass of good red wine. Keeping to this level of acidity is key because it determines a 'healthy' balance of vaginal micro-organisms, or flora, in vaginal mucus."[11]

The acidity in your vagina is necessary to keep it functioning healthfully—don't change it, doctor it, or perfume it; work to embrace it. Similarly, some women report feeling uncomfortable about the fluid or wetness present in the vagina. When women become aroused, lubrication is necessary not only to enjoy sex, but also for sex to be safe. Women become lubricated so that when sex occurs, there is less tearing of the mucosal lining of the vagina. Without lubrication, tearing is more likely to occur, which means you are more vulnerable to STDs.

A necessary prerequisite for becoming comfortable in your own skin is to no longer hate on yourself through cruelly picking at your physical appearance or obsessively doctoring your looks with products and procedures. When women painfully scrutinize their appearance and work to "fix it," they exist in a vigilant state, fearing a flaw will be exposed and feeling awkward, out of sync, and evaluated; all of these qualities make women self-conscious and, as such, are antithetical to pleasurable sex. Studies show that the more preoccupied you are with your physical appearance, the less likely you are to enjoy your sexual experiences.

Part of enjoying your sexuality is developing self-acceptance for your body, just as it is. In order to enjoy sex and to become less self-conscious, work to notice when you are hating on yourself for perceived physical flaws. Find ways to redirect your attention spotlight from physical self-criticism to self-acceptance. No matter what you look like, your body is a vehicle for enjoying the pleasures of life—eating, relaxing, laughing, sleeping, and sex, too. Consider taking up physical activities that make you feel strong and appreciative of what your body can do—yoga, kickboxing, running, martial arts, or dancing. Challenge your negative thoughts about yourself and replace hating on yourself with an appreciation for what your physical body provides you, imperfections and all.

If you are afraid of understanding or becoming comfortable with your sexuality, then how will anyone else learn to please you? A lack of self-understanding and exploration only serves to reinforce the mystery of making women happy and keeps women in the dark about what brings them pleasure.

REFLECT ON YOUR FIRST EXPERIENCES WITH SEX

In order to fully claim your sexuality, it is important to consider your first sexual learning experiences. Just as with emotional development, learning about one's sexuality is based on a pattern that was imprinted early in your development. Consider what you were told as a child about your sexual anatomy and how you learned about the birds and the bees. For example, being told not to touch "down there," or that only bad girls have sex or that you could get a reputation for sleeping around makes girls anxious instead of curious and explorative.

What were you told about sex? What were you told about your body parts? Was shame induced for self-touch? Remember the labels you were taught and what your parents' attitudes were toward your sexuality as well as sex in general. How did your mother and father as individuals react when you were an adolescent and your body was changing? Did they help you to better understand your changing body? Did your parents caution you about guys being out for one thing? Did they take excessive interest in controlling your dress and appearance? Did one or both of your parents begin to notice when you would gain weight? Or did your parents never say anything at all about the birds and the bees or about understanding your changing body?

In addition, each sexual experience you have impacts how competent and capable you feel you are sexually. Your sexual blueprint is developed by your first sexual experiences with romantic partners and then with each subsequent sexual experience over time. This is another reason why it is important to choose your partners thoughtfully.

Review your first learning experiences with sex and consider what themes emerge. Was your sexuality treated with respect in your family, and likewise, do you now pick partners who treat you with respect by making sure you are not judged and that you are well attended to? Or, when you were young, were you told little about your developing sexuality beyond criticism or caution, and likewise, do you now pick partners with whom you feel guarded and judged? Challenge and rework these early learning experiences if upon reflection you see a theme of little information, criticism, and fear instead of openness to your experience of your changing self.

It is important to thoroughly convince yourself that sexual pleasure is a healthy part of your identity. Work toward developing an open-minded, curious, nonjudgmental, physical approach to understanding your sexual self. This approach will allow you to discover your sexual response patterns and what will arouse you.

INCREASE PLEASURE

With so much to do and the pressure to do it all so perfectly, many women do not stop to eat lunch let alone connect with what drives their physical pleasure. In the face of this pressure, women may adopt a get-it-done mentality when it comes to sex and disengage from their in-the-moment experience. Disengaging from pleasure and displeasure partly explains why a woman may pursue unfulfilling and even unsafe sexual experiences.

Build an ability to connect with your sexuality by tuning in to your physical experiences and verbally labeling your likes and dislikes to yourself. Do at least one thing every day that you—not your partner, lover, friend, or child—enjoy. Participate in meditation, use visual imagery, partake in a massage, or find other ways to help you learn to stay connected with physical sensations.

Learn to take pleasure listening to music, sharing a good laugh, and enjoying a delicious meal. Try not to rush through life; allow at least some of your experiences to impact you. Sharpen your awareness for when you are physically uncomfortable, if your pants are too tight, if you are fatigued, if you have a headache, or if you are hungry or thirsty.

Time and again, women report engaging in sex without enjoying the experience and, in some cases, experiencing physical pain. Being your own best caretaker means noticing when you are physically uncomfortable and taking steps to restore your comfort. Consider not proceeding with a sexual encounter unless you have compelling evidence from your experience with the person, through open communication and emotional intimacy, that pleasure will ensue. If you go forward with a particular partner and it becomes physically painful, by all means stop the sexual encounter.

Each time you engage in sex for external reasons, including to gain a relationship, to get a self-esteem boost, or to briefly escape being alone, you deny yourself the opportunity to develop and understand your sexual preferences. Notice when you are disconnecting from a sexual experience and work to stay in your own head. Rather than thinking about your partner's desire, keep your attention spotlight directed toward your physical and mental sensations.

CULTIVATE *YOUR* SEXUAL NARRATIVE

Following a male narrative of sex is typical of many women. These women derive sexual pleasure solely through feeling their partner's desire. As a result of wanting to please in relationships, many women only feel desirable if they are providing sexual pleasure yet become awkward and self-conscious when receiving it. The more prone a woman is to seeing herself through the eyes of her partner, the harder it is for her to know her own pleasure. For women, sexual pleasure occurs not only through understanding the body, but also through knowing what stimulates the mind. In order to enjoy sex, it is important to develop a narrative of what is mentally stimulating to you.

Consider your point of view about sex. What is your narrative for how sex should proceed? Notice your judgments about yourself and others and how these judgments may keep you from fully understanding your sexual self and from having a fulfilling sex life. What is tolerable, intolerable, pleasurable, likable, or uncomfortable in your sexual narrative? Do you believe that sex is to be enjoyed by you, or is it mainly for him? Do you have a narrative that men are just "out for one thing" or are sexual predators? Are women who enjoy sex loose or slutty? Does your pleasure narrative stop with giving your partner pleasure? If you only dwell on cultural stereotypes about men and women, you forgo learning what you desire, and your sexual pleasure will remain elusive.

Take control and responsibility for enjoying your sex life by developing a new sexual narrative that includes your fantasies and preferences. The more you believe you are a sexual being and that sex is an important aspect of your identity, the easier it will be for you to develop a fulfilling and pleasurable sex life. Notice when you are going to the external (how your partners or society view you), and see yourself and your sexual needs and desires separate from judgments and stereotypes.

If you have difficulty feeling comfortable exploring your own body, ask yourself why. What do you fear? What could be more natural than knowing your own body? Why not explore your sexuality independent of others? If you do not take an active interest in understanding your sexual self, how can you expect a partner to find that understanding? Through challenging the roadblocks to your sexual fulfillment, you will liberate yourself to be curious and to fully explore what drives your pleasure.

The remainder of the chapter is devoted to taking this increased knowledge about your sexuality into your romantic relationships. The information provided is meant to help you make well-informed choices about your sexuality.

DON'T DRINK THE KOOL-AID

An interesting phenomenon often presents itself in female sexual development. Some women cope by developing a mentality that says, "If I can't beat them, I am going to join them," and then they work to convince themselves they are "just like men" when it comes to sex. They shun emotional intimacy and declare to themselves, as well as to others, that they only want one thing: good sex. They may tell themselves they are "using" their romantic partners and believe no-strings-attached sex is a way to even out a sexual double standard. This mindset may look tempting on the surface, but ultimately, it is self-defeating.

Drinking this Kool-Aid is an attempt to conquer the sexual contradictions present for women in our culture and represents an understandable quest for independence and freedom. In actuality, this mindset results in blocking that which has the capacity to bring women lasting fulfillment. As explored early on in this book, women thrive in relationships that offer a sense of belonging, acceptance, and authentic connection, as well as avenues to provide and receive nurturance. Although there may be times in a woman's life where casual sex really is casual, most of the time and for most women, sex represents a way in some degree to become emotionally closer to their partners.

Because female identity is formed around relationships and closeness with others, it is nearly impossible, whatever they may tell themselves, for many women to separate bonding and attachment from physical sex. Nevertheless, some blind themselves to signs, obvious to others, that they are attaching to a man—talking about him a great deal, having a strong desire to see him, daydreaming about him, or preferring his company over others. If it is only sex, a woman's focus is exclusively on the physical sensations of the sex act itself with no particular desire to ever see the partner again.

The interesting contradiction is that many of the women I talk to who fall into this dynamic say very little about the thrill of the sexual experience itself. Despite their best efforts, they talk about the guys they hook up with in terms of wanting a more lasting connection. Their focus is not how hot the sex was. They are driven by a strong desire to bond. They seek him out at social events. They find it hard to end encounters with him. They text him or drop by to see him. It is inordinately difficult for women to separate attachment from sexual desire, and there is a biological explanation as to why.

The neurochemicals that are part of the brain's bonding process, including oxytocin, vasopressin, and dopamine, are involved in sexual behavior. Women tend to release greater amounts of oxytocin during sexual activity than men, and the amount released is correlated with orgasm intensity for many women.[12] It is important to be aware of this because oxytocin is widely known to be the brain's bonding chemical. It is released during childbirth and nursing and helps mothers to attach to their infants. Oxytocin provides new mothers with a high that makes them feel good while nursing or while looking into the eyes of their newborns and is one of nature's ways of ensuring that moms are rewarded so they will care for their offspring.

The finding that oxytocin is released for women during sexual experiences means each time you engage in sex, your brain is working to form an attachment to your partner. You are attaching to each person with whom you choose to have sex; even if they are reprehensible as people or ineffective as lovers, you are allowing yourself to bond with them. Sexual pleasure and attachment are inseparable for most women. Despite your best efforts, you may find yourself attaching.

Being your own caretaker means not allowing yourself to forge relationships with men who are unwilling or incapable of meeting your natural need to be cared for and known. Real empowerment is only agreeing to sex with partners who are able to satisfy you and who provide you with some level of safety and emotional intimacy outside of the sex act.

DELAY GRATIFICATION

Women who struggle with sextimacy typically suffer with a depleted self. They may have low self-esteem, body image issues, eating disorders, anxiety, and/or depression. Because they already feel so poorly about themselves, women with low self-esteem are more likely to give in to impulse and ignore long-term risks. They tend to focus on the possibility (no matter how minute) that something positive may occur if they act on impulse. Quite to the contrary, each sextimacy event leaves the woman involved feeling even more depleted and negative about herself than she did prior to the event, which places her at increased risk for yet another sextimacy event.

The most important aspect of taking control of the sextimacy cycle is recognizing that to ensure long-term fulfillment with a romantic partner, you must temporarily forgo acting on the immediate thrill that comes from feeling desirable to men. Allow the excitement to abate so you may eventually find a more meaningful relationship grounded in your best interest.

In a widely known Stanford University study conducted by Walter Mischel,[13] the importance of delayed gratification, or the ability to wait in order to obtain a more desired goal or object, was recognized to be an essential ingredient for healthy child development. In this study, researchers offered young children a marshmallow. Children were told that they could eat the marshmallow immediately, but if they waited fifteen minutes to eat it, they would be given a second marshmallow. The children who were able to wait to eat the marshmallow employed all sorts of creative tactics to distract and not give in to temptation, including singing, closing their eyes, turning around so as not to look at the marshmallow, and using the marshmallow as a toy. Some of the children, on the other hand, ate the marshmallow immediately when the researchers left the room.

In follow-up studies, researchers discovered that those preschool children who delayed gratification for longer periods of time were more competent as adolescents. They were more socially astute and emotionally grounded and performed better academically than those who ate the marshmallow on impulse.

The ability to delay gratification is a skill you can learn to apply to your sexual experiences. To delay gratification, fully articulate to yourself what will fulfill you romantically, without engaging in self-deception. If you believe that you just want casual sex, challenge your expectations and notice whether deep down you think or hope sex might lead to a meaningful relationship.

Remind yourself that research shows most women do not even enjoy sex without emotional intimacy. Remember that every time you engage in sextimacy, you increase your risk of repeating this dynamic, which makes it harder and harder for you to be comfortable with the get-to-know-you process and thus harder to stop substituting hastened sex for intimacy.

Make a conscious choice about your personal policy on sex before you find yourself in a sexual situation and be prepared to remind yourself why this choice is in your long-term best interest. In the event you find yourself swooning for some hot prospect, ask a close friend to help you remember what you can have if you wait to become sexual with this person. When presented with a sextimacy partner, tell yourself that if you "eat the marshmallow," you are sacrificing true intimacy for a short-lived rush of self-esteem that will likely yield little emotional or sexual pleasure.

TAKE THE FLIRT

As you reflect on your personal policy on sex, be mindful of when you are substituting cultural stereotypes about women for your own perspective. Stereotypical examples of reasons for deciding not to engage in a hookup may include fear of being labeled a "slut" or the idea that "good girls take their time in relationships" or "all guys are only out for one thing" or "don't give the milk away for free." These viewpoints may or may not represent good advice, but they have not stopped you in the past. Put them to the side; this is a time to simply consider what, deep down, you want sexually and what is in your best interest. Notice if you are rationalizing or engaging in self-deception to justify a decision that may not be healthy.

Consider the guys in your life, past and present, and how sexual advances are usually presented to you. Think through handling these scenarios in a manner that is different for you in that you maintain your self-respect and long-term goals. When you consider becoming sexual with a particular partner, ask yourself how you will feel about yourself the next day. Will it deepen the connection and help you to feel even closer? Alternatively, will you feel awkward and empty inside? Ask yourself why you wish to have sex—is it a need to feel validated, to find a relationship, or to keep your partners pleased with you? Or do you wish to have sex out of a strong yearning for pleasure, for him as well as for yourself? Consider if you are engaging in sex or a hookup in order to feel better about yourself, to quell loneliness, or perhaps in the hope that sex might turn a causal relationship into a committed one.

Women often report not wishing to turn down a sexual advance from someone they are attracted to out of fear that the rejection will rupture the relationship. However, men typically do not end a relationship because a woman refuses sex; this is actually quite rare. Most men anticipate that they will be turned down sexually and have experienced sexual rejection many times. Men seldom report feeling hurt or upset by women who directly state their sexual comfort level; in fact, most men report that they prefer to know what the women in their lives want when it comes to sex.[14]

If you go forth and have sex with a partner knowing that you may feel worse the next day, then you are intentionally putting yourself in harm's way. Ask yourself why you engage in this self-defeating, masochistic pattern. Are you afraid you cannot handle developing real intimacy? If so, review chapters 4 through 6 in this book and work on strengthening your sense of self. Or are you afraid that you cannot get someone better because you are unworthy or undeserving of lasting fulfillment? If so, work on challenging these beliefs through reflection and noticing when your thoughts are self-defeating or irrational. Remind yourself that happiness is not about deserving or undeserving but, rather, about knowing what you want, believing you can get it, and working to get there.

Are you engaging in sex as a shortcut to the hard work of relationship development and intimacy? There are no shortcuts; if you do not do the work to develop a strong sense of self and to become known by your partners, then you will likely continue to reengage in sextimacy.

If through this reflection you believe having sex with a particular partner is not in your long-term interest, then hold yourself to this. Build relationships with men prior to injecting sex into the mix. Remember that the sex will be more enjoyable later if you simply develop an accepting, open, nonjudgmental way of being together. In the meantime, take the flirt, enjoy male attention while you date, and get to know multiple men without sex. Find ways to enjoy male attention without allowing your relationships to become spoiled by sextimacy.

Notice if you are considering sexual intimacy with a romantic partner out of genuine desire and a wish to deepen the growing emotional bond between you. Become your own best caretaker by only having sex if you actually desire it and if you believe there is enough open communication present for you to receive pleasure. Complete the exercise at the end of this chapter to help you determine whether there is enough emotional intimacy present between you and your partner for a pleasurable sexual experience.

FIND YOUR SEXUAL VOICE

One particularly compelling aspect of the once widely successful television show *Sex and the City* is the ease with which the characters chat openly about their sexuality and about their romantic partners. With the help of so much thoughtful reflection, Carrie, Charlotte, Samantha, and Miranda appear to make deliberate and conscious choices about their sexual experiences. Their predicaments and sexual choices are all considered from a woman's point of view, and cultural stereotypes are openly challenged. The consequences of their sexual experiences (good and bad) are discussed without judgment or shame.

Engaging in open communication with romantic partners as well as male and female friends with whom you can be open and explorative will help you to make thoughtful decisions regarding your sex life. As you communicate about your sexual dilemmas, questions, and insecurities and hear those of others, you will become more comfortable with your sexual voice.

One fantasy that many men and women share is that when sex is with the right partner, it is an easy passion that naturally evolves into uninhibited comfort and ecstasy. When a steamy courtship devolves into unfulfilling sex, both partners often feel disappointed, believing the match must not be a good one. Similarly, many women erroneously hold on to the self-defeating belief that if their sexual partner does not intuitively know how to sexually please, then "he must not really care about me." These women believe that when Mr. Right does come along, he will immediately and magically deliver endless pleasure, thus proving he really must be "the one." Quite to the contrary, wild, uninhibited, orgasmic sex without emotional intimacy is actually a nonexistent experience for most women. The reality is good sex takes self-knowledge and communication. Couples who openly talk about their sexual preferences, desires, needs, turn-ons, and turn-offs have more fulfilling sex lives.

It is likely challenging enough for you to understand your sexuality, let alone for your partner to intuitively know how to please you. In order to enjoy more pleasurable sexual experiences, take responsibility for your own sexual fulfillment by becoming comfortable with direct communication. It is important not only to be able to tell your partner what you like, but also to be open about what you like about him and to be curious about his preferences.

Across the board, open communication about the sex act itself is associated with increased sexual satisfaction for women. When a relationship is just beginning, it is much harder to engage in open dialogue about sexual preferences, as understandably, there is not as much emotional intimacy present. It takes time but feeling comfortable in discussing your sexuality with your partner is a good sign that emotional intimacy is present.

CONCLUSION

For many women, their sexuality is an aspect of self that is sacrificed in order to meet an external standard of desirability. The more you focus on appearing perfectly physically pleasing and coiffed for the men in your life, the more disconnected you become from your experience of pleasure and desire. Fostering a pleasurable sex life with emotional intimacy means learning to know yourself.

SELF-ASSESSMENT: ARE YOU READY TO HAVE SEX WITH THIS POTENTIAL PARTNER?

Take this self-assessment to find out whether you are psychologically and emotionally prepared to become sexual with a particular partner. Answering affirmatively to questions 1 through 10 suggests you are not ready to have sex with this prospect. Answering affirmatively to questions 11 through 20 suggests that emotional intimacy is present for you in this relationship.

1. Do you fear he will be angry with you if you do not agree to sex?
2. Are you considering sex to cement the relationship?
3. Will you feel alone or empty after the encounter is over?
4. Do you imagine your partner will leave soon after the sexual encounter is over?
5. Are you hoping that sex will elicit a commitment from your partner or pull him closer to you?
6. Are you considering becoming sexual early on in your relationship with this person?
7. Do you have sex with guys and then regret it at a later date?
8. Do you fantasize about doing other nonsexual activities with your partner but, in actuality, spend little time together?
9. Do you feel your partner values you, but only when it is convenient for him to do so?
10. Do you feel inhibited and overly concerned about your appearance when in the presence of your partner?

11. Do you truly desire sex and feel aroused when you think of your partner?
12. Are you able to talk with your partner openly about what you like and dislike in your life?
13. Have you enjoyed life together, for example, movies, sunsets, walking, talking, and laughing?
14. Do you consider this a committed relationship?
15. Do you feel known on some level by your partner?
16. Do you feel respected and valued by your partner on a consistent basis?
17. Does your partner take an interest in getting to know how you think and what you like?
18. Do you feel safe with your partner?
19. Are you attracted to and curious about your partner's sexual side?
20. Are you and your partner able to discuss what it would be like to have sex before it occurs?

9

HOUSEKEEPING

Putting It All Together

When you stop to consider the violence and mistreatment women experience the world over, it is no wonder many struggle with low self-esteem and a lost sense of self. The whole world is preoccupied and anxious about female sexuality, and cultures develop primitive ways to manage this discomfort. It is estimated that three million women and girls throughout the world are enslaved in sexual servitude, trapped in brothels and forced to have sex. In Africa, another three million girls undergo female genital mutilation each year. And once every two hours, a woman in India loses her life as a result of bride burning so that her husband is free to remarry or as punishment for an insufficient dowry or some other infraction. According to a study by the World Health Organization, in the majority of countries, 30 to 60 percent of women have at one point experienced sexual or physical violence by a romantic partner.[1] It is estimated in the United States that close to one in five women have been raped in their lifetime, and one in four women has been the victim of physical violence at the hands of a romantic partner.[2]

Mistreatment may begin at conception. Some soon-to-be parents experience disappointment and regret when they learn their baby is a girl. Female babies are more likely than male babies to be aborted or left for dead in some parts of the world. And girls are less likely to be taken to the hospital when they are sick, to receive vaccinations, or to attend school. A 1988 study found that married couples in the United States are less likely to divorce when they have sons than when they have daughters, and if they do divorce, fathers are more likely to maintain custody of their sons than their daughters.[3] It is fair to ask if the same study would show similar trends today, but we should keep in mind that a girl born in 1988 would be twenty-four as I write this.

It is a double whammy when girls grow up without healthy male role models while they are simultaneously sexualized by the culture long before they are cognitively and emotionally prepared. Padded bikini tops, special tennis shoes designed to shape up a tween's derrière, and sparkly eye shadow and lipstick are marketed with pink and purple cartoon characters to attract very young girls. And, amid this barrage, it is difficult for them to develop a multilayered identity or find a firm sense of what they like outside of striving to appear perfectly physically pleasing.

Society warmly invites girls to use their sexuality to gain acceptance and connection, but once they do, they are punished with social judgment and rejection. We see this dynamic play out in girls and adult women taking a highly judgmental view of one another's sexual experiences as well as in low-brow reality shows, such as *Teen Mom* and *16 and Pregnant*. The public's appetite for shaming and humiliating girls who overtly engage in sextimacy or who become pregnant at a young age, outside of marriage, can be sickening to watch. All at once, adolescent girls learn that their sexuality is not only a hot commodity but, surprise, a liability. Fast girls wear a badge of shame; if they become pregnant, that may be the least of their worries.

Girls are repeatedly exposed, through direct experiences and media, to messages that encourage them in dating and marriage to go along to get along because not getting along carries far too much risk. Society's anxiety about female sexuality is turned onto the girls themselves, by making them feel deeply self-conscious about their very girlie-ness. I am dismayed at how often I hear a newly pregnant mom expecting a girl announce that she is nervous or uptight about the "drama" she is in store for from this daughter. As early as conception, some women give their girls negative labels and even a personality that warns all involved to brace for the infant's impact. In this way, these women transfer their own thwarted emotionality onto their daughters, unwittingly creating the very drama they wish to avoid.

Too often our girls are simply left with few internal resources to forge a healthy and empowered sense of self. A recent large-scale survey that included more than two hundred thousand incoming freshman university students found that the percentage of female students who rate their emotional health as below average is at an all-time high and significantly higher than that of male students.[4] The degree of discouragement felt by some women means that for them, it can seem easier to adapt and become part of what bridles than to make significant changes. All of which contributes to women believing there is little they can do to alter their circumstances.

To get what you truly desire from your relationships, begin the process of genuinely and thoroughly attending to yourself. If you do not value yourself, no one else will show you the loving care you need. Housekeeping is the work of tending to your sense of self. Self-awareness and self-acceptance are necessary ingredients for a solid sense of self and for developing healthy relationships. Keeping your own house in order includes thoughtful reflection on that which you truly desire and a belief that, if you are determined, you can get what you want.

EMOTIONAL INTIMACY IS NOT EMOTIONAL DEPENDENCY

There are no shortcuts; only you can build your sense of self. Emotional intimacy with a partner is grounded in your ability to understand your own emotional reactions. Emotional dependency is when you believe someone else can somehow learn to know you when you do not know yourself. If you cannot function or manage your emotional world on your own, then attempts at emotional intimacy in relationships are futile. Intimacy with another is a back-and-forth process of mutual nurturing and communication based on genuine interest. Emotional intimacy is not using your romantic partners or friends as emotional receptacles, where you dump your negative emotion while expecting them to put you back together again. In order for others to feel close to you, they cannot feel perpetually burdened by your needs.

Make the effort to become fully aware of your ongoing emotional reactions to the people and events in your life. As you attend to your experiences, through observing and labeling your emotional reactions, you will find you have more options for gaining control over your weaknesses. If you choose to internalize your negative emotions, then the problematic love patterns you experience in relationships will continue. Self-reflect and notice when you are rationalizing away your feelings. Allow your feelings airtime, at least within your own head, because they reveal how you are actually experiencing your life and what you need for contentment.

VALUE YOURSELF

Many women exist in a world where they do not see their value and learn only to value themselves when others do. These women work to feel valued by pleasing others to the exclusion of their own feelings. The more you view others' mistreatment of you as something you have the ability to fix, tweak, or amend, the harder it is to develop a positive sense of yourself. Seeing yourself exclusively through the eyes of others disconnects you from your day-to-day, moment-to-moment experience of your life.

When you have an urge to dress up negative feelings about yourself, slow down and look at how you are feeling deep within your core. Instead of obscuring your insecurities with men, stop and reflect on what it is you struggle to accept within yourself. Gently remind yourself that you are a worthwhile person and that no one is immune from flaws. Notice how you speak to yourself in your own head about your imperfections. Adopt a loving and compassionate way of acknowledging what you feel poorly about and accept yourself as you are.

As opposed to generally feeling bad about yourself, consider whether you can find specific areas of growth to improve upon. For example, instead of saying, "I suck at relationships," or "No one is ever going to love me," develop awareness for the emotional baggage you carry into your relationships. Then list specific opportunities for growth, for example: managing conflict or developing a middle-ground way of both expressing your needs and tolerating differences.

Challenge yourself with new relationships and experiences that do not come easily to you. Be persistent about approaching these experiences differently. When you do have a setback, search for what you might do differently the next time.

Turn down the volume on self-consciousness, repetitive anxieties, and negative thoughts by filling your life with experiences and relationships that are meaningful and give you a sense of purpose. Do not neglect the basics. Recognize that self-esteem is improved by allowing yourself to do simple, daily rituals that help you to feel a healthy sense of control—eating well, exercising, accomplishing goals, self-reflection, and connecting with the larger world around you. You must determinedly show yourself that you value yourself most of all.

MAKE FULLY AWARE CHOICES

Recognize that each time you choose to engage a new partner sexually, you also are choosing to attach to him. This means that even if you do not really like the guy, and even if he is emotionally stunted, intellectually dull, or sexually inadequate, you are still forming a connection with him. This connection impacts how positively or negatively you see yourself and how capable you believe you are to get what you want romantically. When sextimacy repeats, an opportunity to grow is lost. For you to achieve the happiness you seek, your brain needs to be challenged with new and healthy relationship experiences.

You can have emotional intimacy and erotic sex with the same person, but to accomplish this, you must assess your partners deliberately and choose thoughtfully. Learn to recognize your own desire and notice if, when, and with whom you truly wish to pursue a sexual encounter. Make a commitment to yourself to not engage in any relationship or sexual activity that is not an authentic representation of what you desire. Engaging partners with whom you are self-conscious and insecure will backfire. When there is no emotional intimacy present, sex is not pleasurable for most women, and yet, perversely, biology leads them to feelings of attachment.

Although it is normal and even healthy to want to experiment sexually, do so with your eyes wide open. If you choose a person who is essentially a stranger, be sure your expectations match reality. Every time you consider engaging sexually with a partner, stop to reflect on your innermost feelings, your long-term goals, and your ultimate best interest.

TAKE YOUR RELATIONSHIPS SERIOUSLY

A popular idea holds that in order to have a solid romantic relationship, you must first work alone on self-improvement—"I just need to do me for a while," or "I am cutting myself off from dating until I get myself together." In my experience, when women do this, they often banish themselves to an arbitrary exile, where they feel sad and out of touch. With such a vague goal of "working on myself," self-enlightenment eludes and despair compounds, often culminating in another round of sextimacy. Working on yourself through developing greater self-understanding, self-esteem, and direct communication does not occur in a vacuum. You need your relationships with romantic partners, as well as your friendships, in order to truly know yourself. Each dating experience provides you with in-the-moment data about your preferences, your weaknesses, and your strengths.

Take all of your relationships seriously. It is not contradictory to be self-sufficient and independent while valuing your relationships for providing important aspects of contentment and wellbeing. Allow yourself to participate fully in your relationships; learn from your successes and disappointments. Give in to your healthy need for love, while knowing that you are strong enough to survive, come what may. You are not a sappy female stereotype if you experience heartbreak and sadness over a relationship loss. It is human to have those feelings.

At the same time, explore what drives you separate from your intimate relationships. What kind of work, creative contributions, and humanitarian initiatives give you a sense of accomplishment and fulfillment? Developing an interest, outside of intimate relationships, singlehandedly increases self-esteem and decreases depression for women. And it will make you resilient during the dating process. Find a place where you feel useful, in control, and competent that has nothing to do with attracting men or pleasing others. Endeavor to develop a lasting sense of meaning and purpose through forging connections with the world around you.

SHOUT IT FROM YOUR MEGAPHONE

The status quo can be changed: If sextimacy is not what you want, stop enabling it. The hookup culture is fraught with problems. Women embrace it because they feel it is the only show in town. In the process, many settle for a fraction of what they actually desire. Sextimacy for some presents an easy but profoundly insular way of connecting with men because the true self need not be revealed. When she circumvents the toil of relationship building, a woman places her feelings in a box and does not invest her real self in the union.

There is no substitute for knowing yourself and communicating who you are to your romantic partners. Use your ability to communicate to let the men in your life know what you expect and need to be happy. Be real with yourself about what it is you really want and, then, directly talk with potential partners about your wishes. Language is power, yet many otherwise articulate women suppress this resource when communicating with a romantic partner. Conversation is the pathway to emotional intimacy.

In my work, I find that when women become completely honest with themselves, most of them want emotional intimacy. If this is your goal—a sexually fulfilling, intimate, loving relationship—then own it. Recognizing that you need a committed relationship with someone who truly wants to know the real you does not make you weak; it makes you healthy. If you want love, only you can slow down the relationship-building process enough to get it. Once you know what it is you really want and what will ultimately bring you a satisfying life, say it clearly, and say it often.

As I approached the end of this book, one of my clients, sixteen-year-old Anna, came into my office one day. Anna giggled and smiled as she spoke, her hair in two ponytails, looking every bit the combination of a little girl and a grown woman. A recent breakup with a boyfriend and resulting negative feelings about herself catapulted Anna from a “good girl” to a “bad girl.” Within a matter of weeks, she filled the sadness and heartache with a steady diet of hookups. She chose partners who were at best superficially interested in her, or as she described them, "caring assholes." When I asked her what she liked about hooking up, she said it felt exciting and nodded eagerly when I added "like a rush." I asked if she could enjoy being desired without having sex, and she responded that she could never stop herself at that point. When I suggested that she could still have a steamy encounter without sex, and that it might even add to the allure, she laughed me off. I tried again, "Maybe you could draw it out a little, even a day or so, just to make sure your feelings are on board?" Anna looked at me as if I had two heads and giggled at my suggestions.

In particular, Anna was quite interested in hooking up with Tyler, who continued to give her the cold shoulder. She wanted to seek him out, made efforts to speak with him, and worked on appearing as desirable as possible when she knew she would be in his presence. He sometimes gave her a grunt or a "lookin' good" when she walked by, but otherwise, he was aloof and disinterested. Nonetheless, Anna pursued him and worked to be in his vicinity as much as possible.

I finally asked her, "What is it about Tyler, a guy who doesn't even give you a 'hi' much less a 'how are you,' that keeps you putting all of your energy into trying to please him?" She looked at me knowingly, as if to say, "Isn't it so frickin' obvious?", paused and then explained: "You know, it's the don't-give-a-shit attitude—we, women, always like the bad boys, ya know what I mean?" Although I did know what she meant, I wanted to hear it articulated.

I pushed: "Yes, I know the stereotype, but can you tell me what it is about the 'bad boy' that appeals to you?" She thought for a moment and said, "You know, he's the guy with attitude, swagger, like he doesn't need anything, he's always in control . . . he seems like he doesn't have a care in the world, and if you can make him care about you, then you must be the shit. You just think, someday, he'll want me, and then I'll know I am on my game."

And there it was, clearly stated. If you can make he who cares so little care, then you must be a worthwhile person. I pushed some more, "But what about what *you* think of you?" Anna laughed me off as naïve and overfeeling. She did listen as I explained sextimacy and how it erodes self-esteem and how, for many women, it is a self-defeating attempt to gain what truly satisfies. Noticing her discomfort with the topic, I ended it by asking her merely to stop to think for a moment about what she wants each time she finds herself drawn to another sextimacy event. She responded by changing directions in the conversation, and we pursued a new topic. We said our goodbyes, and she left. A few minutes later, Anna popped her head back in my office. The giggles and smile were gone. In their place was a serious, thoughtful young woman. "Alright, I'll think about it."

Bibliography

ABC's *20/20* Investigation into what keeps the franchise booming, March 2010. Retrieved from http://xfinity.comcast.net/blogs/tv/2010/03/16/the-bachelor-a-behind-the-scenes-look-at-calculated-drama.

Ainsworth, M., Blehar, M., Waters, E., & Wall, S. (1979). *Patterns of attachment.* New York: Psychology Press.

Alexander, B. (2010, June 30). "Sorry guys: Up to 80 percent of women admit faking it." *Sexploration on NBCNews.com.* Retrieved from http://www.msnbc.msn.com/id/38006774/ns/health-sexual_health/t/sorry-guys-percent-women-admit-faking-it.

Allgood-Merten, B., Lewinsohn, P. M., & Hops, H. (1990). Sex differences in adolescent depression. *Journal of Abnormal Psychology, 99*, 55–63.

Babcock, J., Waltz, J., Jacobson, N., & Gottman, J. (1993). Power and violence: The relation between communication patterns, power discrepancies, and domestic violence. *Journal of Consulting and Clinical Psychology, 61*, 40–50.

Barlow, D. H. (1988). *Anxiety and its disorders: The nature and treatment of anxiety and panic* (1st ed.). New York: Guilford Press.

Bavelier, D., Dye, M., & Hauser, P. C. (2006). Do deaf individuals see better? *Trends in Cognitive Sciences, 10*, 512–518.

Blackledge, C. (2003). *The story of V: A natural history of female sexuality.* New Brunswick, NJ: Rutgers University Press.

Blanchard-Fields, F., Sulsky, L., & Robinson-Whelen, S. (1991). Moderating effects of age and context on the relationship between gender, sex role differences, and coping. *Sex Roles, 25*, 645–660.

Bliss T., & Lomo, T. (1973). Long-lasting potentiation of synaptic transmission in the dentate area of the anaesthetized rabbit following stimulation of the perforant path. *The Journal of Physiology, 232*, 331–356.

Bogle, K. (2008). *Hooking up: Sex, dating, and relationships on campus.* New York: New York University Press.

Bowlby, J. (1988). *A secure base: Parent-child attachment and healthy human development.* New York: Basic Books.

Breath holding spell (n.d.). In *Medline Plus*. Retrieved from http://www.nlm.nih.gov/medlineplus/ency/article/000967.htm.

Breath holding spells (n.d.). In *Senders Pediatrics*. Retrieved from http://www.senderspediatrics.com/HealthTopics/Health_Topics_A_Z/Behavioral_Emotional_Concerns/Breath_Holding_Spells.page.

Brewer, G., & Hendrie, C. (2011). Evidence to suggest that copulatory vocalizations in women are not a reflexive consequence of orgasm. *Archives of Sexual Behavior, 40*, 559–564.

Brody, L. (1999). *Gender, emotion, and the family.* Cambridge, MA: Harvard University Press.

Brown, K. W., & Ryan, R. M. (2003). The benefits of being present: Mindfulness and its role in psychological well-being. *Journal of Personality and Social Psychology, 84*, 822–848.

Brown, L. M. (2003). *Girlfighting: Betrayal and rejection among girls.* New York: New York University Press.

Brown, L. M., & Gilligan, C. (1992). *Meeting at the crossroads: Women's psychology and girls' development.* Cambridge, MA: Harvard University Press.

Brumberg, J. J. (1997). *The body project: An intimate history of American girls.* New York: Random House.

Burleson, B. R. (1997). Similarities in social skills, interpersonal attraction, and the development of personal relationships. In J. S. Trent (Ed.), *Communication: Views from the helm for the twenty-first century* (77–84). Boston: Allyn & Bacon.

Calkins, S. D., & Johnson, M. C. (1998). Toddler regulation of distress to frustrating events: Temperamental and maternal correlates. *Infant Behavior and Development, 21*, 379–395.

Centers for Disease Control and Prevention (2010, June 4). *Morbidity and mortality weekly report, 55*(5). Retrieved from http://www.cdc.gov/mmwr/pdf/ss/ss5905.pdf.

Centers for Disease Control and Prevention (2011, November). *The national intimate partner and sexual violence survey (NISVS): 2010 summary report.* Retrieved from http://www.cdc.gov/violenceprevention/nisvs/index.html.

Clark, L. A., & Watson, D. (1991). Tripartite model of anxiety and depression: Psychometric evidence and taxonomic implications. *Journal of Abnormal Psychology, 100*, 316–336.

Cole, P. M. (1986). Children's spontaneous control of facial expression. *Child Development, 57*, 1309–1321.

Cozolino, L. (2006). *The neuroscience of human relationships: Attachment and the developing social brain.* New York: W. W. Norton.

Crick, N. R. (1995). Relational aggression: The role of intent attributions, feelings of distress, and provocation type. *Development and Psychopathology, 7*, 313–322.

Crick, N. R., & Werner, N. E. (1998). Response decision processes in relational and overt aggression. *Child Development, 69*, 1630–1639.

Darwin, C. (2004). *The autobiography of Charles Darwin*. Charleston, SC: BookSurge Classics.

Daubman, K., & Sigall, H. (1997). Gender differences in perceptions of how others are affected by self-disclosure of achievement. *Sex Roles, 37*, 73–89.

Davis, T. L. (1995). Gender differences in masking negative emotions: Ability or motivation? *Developmental Psychology, 31*, 660–667.

Denham, S., Bassett, H. H., & Wyatt, T. (2008). The socialization of emotional competence. In J. Grusec & P. Hastings (Eds.), *Handbook of socialization* (614–637). New York: Guilford Press.

Diamond, L. M. (2004). Emerging perspectives on distinctions between romantic love and sexual desire. *Current Directions in Psychological Science, 13*, 116–119.

Driesen, N., & Raz, N. (1995). The influence of sex, age, and handedness on corpus callosum morphology: A meta-analysis. *Psychobiology, 23*, 240–247.

Dunn, J., Bretherton, I., & Munn, P. (1987). Conversations about feeling states between mothers and their children. *Developmental Psychology, 23*, 132–139.

Durham, M. G. (2008). *The Lolita effect: The media sexualization of young girls and what we can do about it*. New York: Overlook Press.

Dutton, D. G., & Aron, A. P. (1974). Some evidence for heightened sexual attraction under conditions of high anxiety. *Journal of Personality and Social Psychology, 30*, 510–517.

Dweck, C. S. (2000). *Self-theories: Their role in motivation, personality, and development*. New York: Psychology Press.

Dweck, C. S. (2006). *Mindset: The new psychology of success*. New York: Random House.

Eriksson, P. S., Perfilieva, E., Björk-Eriksson, T., Alborn, A. M., Nordborg, C., Peterson, D. A., & Gage, F. H. (1998). Neurogenesis in the adult hippocampus. *Nature Medicine, 4*, 1313–1317.

Etxebarria, I., Ortiz, M. J., Conejero, S., & Pascual, A. (2009). Intensity of habitual guilt in men and women: Differences in interpersonal sensitivity and the tendency towards anxious-aggressive guilt. *Spanish Journal of Psychology, 12*, 540–554.

Falbo, T., & Peplau, L. A. (1980). Power strategies in intimate relationships. *Journal of Personality and Social Psychology, 38*, 618–628.

Fletcher, G., & Simpson, J. A. (2000). Ideal standards in close relationships: Their structure and functions. *Directions in Psychological Science, 9*, 102–105.

Ford, M. B., & Collins, N. L. (2010). Self-esteem moderates neuroendocrine and psychological responses to interpersonal rejection. *Journal of Personality and Social Psychology, 98*, 405–419.

Fredrickson, B. L. (2004). The broaden-and-build theory of positive emotions. *Philosophical Transactions of the Royal Society of London, B, Biological Sciences, 359*, 1367–1378.

Giles, H., & Wiemann, J. M. (1987). Language, social comparison, and power. In C. Berger & S. H. Chafee (Eds.), *Handbook of communication science*. Thousand Oaks, CA: Sage.

Gilligan, C. (1982). *In a different voice: Psychological theory and women's development*. Cambridge, MA: Harvard University Press.

Gilligan, C. (2002). *The birth of pleasure*. New York: Alfred A. Knopf.

Glick, P. (1988). Fifty years of family demography: A record of social change. *Journal of Marriage and the Family, 50*, 861–873.

Goleman, D. (1995). *Emotional intelligence*. New York: Bantam Books.

Gottman, J. M. (1999). *The seven principles for making marriage work*. New York: Three Rivers Press.

Gross, E. F. (2009). Logging on, bouncing back: An experimental investigation of online communication following social exclusion. *Developmental Psychology, 45*, 1787–1793.

Gross, J. J. (2002). Emotional regulation: Affective, cognitive, and social consequences. *Psychophysiology, 39*, 281–291.

Gross, J. J., & Thompson, R. A. (2007). Emotion regulation conceptual foundations. In J. J. Gross (Ed.)., *Handbook of emotion regulation* (3–24). New York: Guilford Press.

Guerrero, L. K., Andersen, P. A., & Afifi, W. A. (2011). *Close encounters: Communication in relationships*. Thousand Oaks, CA: Sage Publications.

Guttmacher Institute (February 2012). *Facts on American teens' sources of information about sex*. Retrieved from http://www.guttmacher.org/pubs/FB-Teen-Sex-Ed.html.

Hebb, D. O. (1949). *The organization of behavior: A neuropsychological theory*. New York: Psychology Press.

Hines, M. (2005). *Brain gender*. New York: Oxford University Press.

Holley, S. R., Sturm, V. E., & Levenson, R. W. (2010). Exploring the basis for gender differences in the demand-withdraw pattern. *Journal of Homosexuality, 57*, 666–684.

Huston, T. L., Niehuis, S., & Smith, S. E. (2001). The early marital roots of conjugal distress and divorce. *Directions in Psychological Science, 10*, 116–119.

Iaccino, J. (1993). *Left brain-right brain differences: Inquiries, evidence, and new approaches*. New York: Psychology Press.

Indiana University Medical Center (2006). *Archives of pediatrics and adolescent medicine*. Retrieved from http://www.msnbc.msn.com/id/14169056/ns/health-sexual_health/t/report-many-teens-dont-use-condoms.

John, O. P., & Gross, J. J. (2004). Healthy and unhealthy emotion regulation: Personality processes, individual differences, and life-span development. *Journal of Personality, 72*, 1301–1333.

Kagan, J. (1999). The role of parents in children's psychological development. *Pediatrics, 104*, 164–167.

Kang, S. M., & Shaver, P. R. (2004). Individual differences in emotional complexity: Their psychological implications. *Journal of Personality, 72*, 687–726.

Kenneally, C. (2007). *The first word: The search for the origins of language*. London: Penguin Books.

Kilbourne, J. (1999). *Can't buy my love: How advertising changes the way we think and feel.* New York: Simon & Schuster.

Knee, C. R. (1998). Implicit theories of relationships: Assessment and prediction of romantic relationship initiation, coping, and longevity. *Journal of Personality and Social Psychology, 74*, 360–370.

Kristof, N. D., & WuDunn, S. (2010). *Half the sky: Turning oppression into opportunity for women worldwide.* New York: Vintage.

Laumann, E. O., Paik, A., & Rosen, R. C. (1999). Sexual dysfunction in the United States: Prevalence and predictors. *Journal of the American Medical Association, 281*, 537–544.

Laumann, E. O., Paik, A., Glasser, D. B., Kang, J. H., Wang, T., Levinson, B., Moreira, E. D., Nicolosi, A., & Gingell, C. (2006). A cross-national study of subjective sexual well-being among older women and men: Findings from the global study of sexual attitudes and behaviors. *Archives of Sexual Behavior, 35*, 145–161.

LeDoux, J. (1996). *The emotional brain.* New York: Simon & Schuster.

LeDoux, J. (2002). *The synaptic self.* London: Penguin Books.

Lee, J. A. (1977). A typology of styles of loving. *Personality and Social Psychology Bulletin, 3*, 173–182.

Lehrer, J. (2010, February 25). Depression's upside. *New York Times.* Retrieved from http://www.nytimes.com/2010/02/28/magazine/28depression-t.html?pagewanted=all.

Leith, K. P., & Baumeister, R. F. (1996). Why do bad moods increase self-defeating behavior? Emotion, risk-taking, and self-regulation. *Journal of Personality and Social Psychology, 71*, 1250–1267.

Lennon, R., & Eisenberg, N. (1987). Gender and age differences in empathy and sympathy. In N. Eisenberg and J. Strayer (Eds.), *Empathy and its development.* Cambridge, MA: Cambridge University Press.

Lewin, T. (2011, January 26). Record level of stress found in college freshmen. *New York Times.* Retrieved from http://www.nytimes.com/2011/01/27/education/27colleges.html.

Lewis, T. Amini, F., & Lannon, R. (2000). *A general theory of love.* Random House: New York.

Linehan, M. M. (1993a). *Cognitive-behavioral treatment of borderline personality disorder.* New York: Guilford Press.

Linehan, M. M. (1993b). *Skills training manual for treating borderline personality disorder.* New York: Guilford Press.

Linehan, M. M., Bohus, M., & Lynch, T. R. (2007). Dialectical behavior therapy for pervasive emotion dysregulation. In J. J. Gross (Ed.), *Handbook of emotion regulation* (581–605). New York: Guilford Press.

Lomo, T. (1966). Frequency potentiation of excitatory synaptic activity in the dentate area of the hippocampal formation. *Acta Physiologica Scandinavica 68*(277), 128.

McCleneghan, J. S. (2003). Selling sex to college females: Their attitudes about *Cosmopolitan* and *Glamour* magazines. *Social Science Journal, 40*, 317–325.

Miller, S. L., & Maner, J. K. (2009). Sex differences in response to sexual versus emotional infidelity: The moderating role of individual differences. *Personality and Individual Differences, 46*, 287–291.

Motley, M. T., & Reeder, H. M. (1995). Unwanted escalation of sexual intimacy: Male and female perceptions of connotations and relational consequences of resistance messages. *Communication Monographs, 62*, 355–382.

Nolen-Hoeksema, S., & Jackson, B. (2001). Mediators of the gender difference in rumination. *Psychology of Women Quarterly, 25*, 37–47.

Nolen-Hoeksema, S., Larson, J., & Grayson, C. (1999). Explaining the gender difference in depressive symptoms. *Journal of Personality and Social Psychology, 77*, 1061–1072.

Nolen-Hoeksema, S., Parker, L. E., & Larson, J. (1994). Ruminative coping with depressed mood following loss. *Journal of Personality and Social Psychology, 67*, 92–104.

Ornstein, R. (1991). *The evolution of consciousness: The origins of the way we think.* New York: Prentice-Hall.

Owen, W. F. (1987). The verbal expression of love by women and men as a critical communication event in personal relationships. *Women's Studies in Communication, 10*, 15–24.

Parker-Pope, T. (2008, October 27). Love, sex, and the changing landscape of infidelity. *New York Times*. Retrieved from http://www.nytimes.com/2008/10/28/health/28well.html.

Pipher, M. (1994). *Reviving Ophelia: Saving the selves of adolescent girls*. New York: Ballantine Books.

Plutchik, R. (2002). *Emotions and life: Perspectives from psychology, biology, and evolution*. Washington, DC: American Psychological Association.

Rabin, R. (2011, December 14). Nearly 1 in 5 women in U.S. survey say they have been sexually assaulted. *New York Times*. Retrieved from http://www.nytimes.com/2011/12/15/health/nearly-1-in-5-women-in-us-survey-report-sexual-assault.html.

Radke-Yarrow, M., & Kochanska, G. (1990). Anger in young children. In N. Stein, B. Leventhal, and T. Trabasso (Eds.), *Psychological and biological approaches to emotion*. New York: Psychology Press.

Reis, H. T., & Collins, W. A. (2004). Relationships, human behavior, and psychological science. *Current Directions in Psychological Science, 13*, 233–237.

Reitz, S. (2010, March 29). 9 Charged with Bullying Mass. Teen who Killed Self. Associated Press. Retrieved from http://www.boston.com/news/education/k_12/articles/2010/03/29/9_charged_with_bullying_mass_teen_who_killed_self.

Rosen, W. D., Adamson, L. B., & Bakeman, R. (1992). An experimental investigation of infant social referencing: Mothers' messages and gender differences. *Developmental Psychology, 28*, 1172–1178.

Russell, G., & Russell, A. (1987). Mother-child and father-child relationships in middle childhood. *Child Development, 58*, 1573–1585.

Sadalla, E. K., Kenrick, D. T., & Vershure, B. (1987). Dominance and heterosexual attraction. *Journal of Personality and Social Psychology, 52*, 730–738.

Shoda, Y., Mischel, W., & Peake, P. K. (1990). Predicting adolescent cognitive and self-regulatory competencies from preschool delay of gratification: Identifying diagnostic conditions. *Developmental Psychology, 26*, 978–986.

Simmons, R. (2002). *Odd girl out: The hidden culture of aggression in girls.* New York: Harcourt.

Stegge, H., & Terwogt, M. M. (2007). Awareness and regulation of emotion in typical and atypical development. In J. J. Gross (Ed.), *Handbook of emotion regulation* (269–286). New York: Guilford Press.

Stern, S. T. (2007). *Instant identity.* New York: Peter Lang.

Tamir, M., John, O. P., Srivastava, S., & Gross, J. J. (2007). Implicit theories of emotion: Affective and social outcomes across a major life transition. *Journal of Personality and Social Psychology, 92*, 731–744.

Tangney, J. P. (1995). Shame and guilt in interpersonal relationships. In J. P. Tangney & K. W. Fischer (Eds.), *Self-conscious emotions: The psychology of shame, guilt, embarrassment and pride* (114–139). New York: Guilford Press.

Taylor, S. E. (1983). Adjustment to threatening events: A theory of cognitive adaptation. *American Psychologist, 38*, 1161–1173.

Timmers, M., Fischer, A. H., & Manstead, A. S. R. (1998). Gender differences in motives for regulating emotion. *Personality and Social Psychology Bulletin, 24*, 974–985.

Tolhuizen, J. H. (1989). Communication strategies for intensifying dating relationships: Identification, use, and structure. *Journal of Social and Personal Relationships, 6*, 413–434.

Tolman, D. L. (2002). *Dilemmas of desire: Teenage girls talk about sexuality.* Cambridge, MA: Harvard University Press.

Weissman, M., Bland, R. C., Canino, G. J., Faravelli, C., Greenwald, S., Hwu, H. G., Joyce, P. R., & Yeh, E. K. (1996). Cross-national epidemiology of major depression and bipolar disorder. *Journal of the American Medical Association, 276*, 293–299.

Wenzlaff, R. M., & Wegner, D. M. (2000). Thought suppression. *Annual Review of Psychology, 51*, 59–91.

Wenzlaff, R., Wegner, D. M., & Roper, D. (1988). Depression and mental control: The resurgence of unwanted negative thoughts. *Journal of Personality and Social Psychology, 55*, 882–892.

Wolf, N. (1991). *The beauty myth: How images of beauty are used against women.* New York: William Morrow.

NOTES

CHAPTER 2: PERFECT LITTLE DOLLS

1. Brumberg, J. J. (1997). *The body project: An intimate history of American girls.* New York: Random House.

2. See Gilligan, C. (1982). *In a different voice: Psychological theory and women's development.* Cambridge, MA: Harvard University Press.

3. Brumberg, J. J. (1997). *The body project: An intimate history of American girls.* New York: Random House.

4. Tolman, D. L. (2002). *Dilemmas of desire: Teenage girls talk about sexuality.* Cambridge, MA: Harvard University Press.

5. Tolman, D. L. (2002). *Dilemmas of desire: Teenage girls talk about sexuality.* Cambridge, MA: Harvard University Press.

6. Simmons, R. (2002). *Odd girl out: The hidden culture of aggression in girls* (p. 16). New York: Harcourt.

7. Simmons, R. (2002). *Odd girl out: The hidden culture of aggression in girls* (p. 46). New York: Harcourt.

8. Reitz, S. (2010, March 29). 9 charged with bullying Mass. teen who killed self. Associated Press. Retrieved from http://www.boston.com/news/education/k_12/articles/2010/03/29/9_charged_with_bullying_mass_teen_who_killed_self.

9. Simmons, R. (2002). *Odd girl out: The hidden culture of aggression in girls* (p. 115). New York: Harcourt.

10. For more on the power of healthy female relationships, see Pipher, M. (1994). *Reviving Ophelia: Saving the selves of adolescent girls.* New York: Ballantine Books. See also Brown, L. M., & Gilligan, C. (1992). *Meeting at the crossroads: Women's psychology and girls' development.* Cambridge, MA: Harvard University Press.

11. Brumberg, J. J. (1997). *The body project: An intimate history of American girls.* New York: Random House.

12. Brumberg, J. J. (1997). Perfect skin. In *The body project: An intimate history of American girls.* New York: Random House. (Chapter 3, text from picture 9.)

13. Kilbourne, J. (1999). *Can't buy my love: How advertising changes the way we think and feel.* New York: Simon & Schuster.

14. Kilbourne, J. (1999). *Can't buy my love: How advertising changes the way we think and feel* (p. 145). New York: Simon & Schuster.

15. Durham, M. G. (2008). *The Lolita effect: The media sexualization of young girls and what we can do about it.* Woodstock, NY: Overlook Press.

16. McCleneghan, J. S. (2003). Selling sex to college females: Their attitudes about *Cosmopolitan* and *Glamour* magazines. *Social Science Journal, 40,* 317–325.

17. McCleneghan, J. S. (2003). Selling sex to college females: Their attitudes about *Cosmopolitan* and *Glamour* magazines. *Social Science Journal, 40,* 317–325.

18. Kilbourne, J. (1999). *Can't buy my love: How advertising changes the way we think and feel.* New York: Simon & Schuster.

19. ABC's *20/20* Investigation into what keeps the franchise booming, March 2010. Retrieved from http://xfinity.comcast.net/blogs/tv/2010/03/16/the-bachelor-a-behind-the-scenes-look-at-calculated-drama.

20. Durham, M. G. (2008). *The Lolita effect: The media sexualization of young girls and what we can do about it.* Woodstock, NY: Overlook Press. See also Wolf, N. (1991). *The beauty myth: How images of beauty are used against women.* New York: William Morrow.

21. Kilbourne, J. (1999). *Can't buy my love: How advertising changes the way we think and feel* (p. 261). New York: Simon & Schuster.

22. Tolman, D. L. (2002). *Dilemmas of desire: Teenage girls talk about sexuality* (p. 139). Cambridge, MA: Harvard University Press.

23. Bogle, K. (2008). *Hooking up: Sex, dating, and relationships on campus.* New York University Press.

24. Tolman, D. L. (2002). *Dilemmas of desire: Teenage girls talk about sexuality* (p. 5). Cambridge, MA: Harvard University Press.

25. Tolman, D. L. (2002). *Dilemmas of desire: Teenage girls talk about sexuality* (p. 21). Cambridge, MA: Harvard University Press.

26. Tolman, D. L. (2002). *Dilemmas of desire: Teenage girls talk about sexuality* (p. 129). Cambridge, MA: Harvard University Press.

27. Parker-Pope, T. (2008, October 27). Love, sex and the changing landscape of infidelity. *New York Times.* Retrieved from www.nytimes.com/2008/10/28/health/28well.html. See also http://www.asylum.com/2010/02/25/dr-helen-fisher-biological-anthropologist-on-cheating-adultery.

CHAPTER 3: SUGAR, SPICE, ALL THINGS NICE

1. Iaccino, J. F. (1993). *Left brain–right brain differences: Inquiries, evidence, and new approaches.* New York: Psychology Press.

2. Hines, M. (2005). *Brain gender.* New York: Oxford University Press.

3. Driesen, N., & Raz, N. (1995). The influence of sex, age, and handedness on corpus callosum morphology: A meta-analysis. *Psychobiology, 23*, 240–247.

4. Dunn, J., Bretherton, I., & Munn, P. (1987). Conversations about feeling states between mothers and their young children. *Developmental Psychology, 23*, 132–139.

5. Russell, G., & Russell, A. (1987). Mother-child and father-child relationships in middle childhood. *Child Development, 58*, 1573–1585.

6. Rosen, W. D., Adamson, L. B., & Bakeman, R. (1992). An experimental investigation of infant social referencing: Mothers' messages and gender differences. *Developmental Psychology, 28*, 1172–1178.

7. Cole, P. (1986). Children's spontaneous control of facial expression. *Child Development, 57*, 1309–1321. And Davis, T. L. (1995). Gender differences in masking negative emotions: Ability or motivation? *Developmental Psychology, 31*, 660–667.

8. Radke-Yarrow, M., & Kochanska, G. (1990). Anger in young children. In N. Stein, A. B. Leventhal, and T. Trabasso (Eds.), *Psychological and biological approaches to emotion* (pp. 297–310). Hillsdale, NJ: Erlbaum.

9. Brody, L. (1999). *Gender, emotion, and the family*. Cambridge, MA: Harvard University Press.

10. Pipher, M. (1994). *Reviving Ophelia: Saving the selves of adolescent girls*. New York: Ballantine.

11. Gilligan, C. (2002). *The birth of pleasure*. New York: Alfred A. Knopf.

12. Allgood-Mertin, B., Lewinsohn, P. M., & Hops, H. (1990). Sex differences in adolescent depression. *Journal of Abnormal Psychology, 99*, 55–63. Also see Blanchard-Fields, F., Sulsky, L., & Robinson-Whelen, S. (1991). Moderating effects of age and context on the relationship between gender, sex role differences, and coping. *Sex Roles, 25*, 645–660. Nolen-Hoeksema, S., Larson, J., & Grayson, C. (1999). Explaining the gender difference in depressive symptoms. *Journal of Personality and Social Psychology, 77*, 1061–1072. Nolen-Hoeksema, S., Parker, L. E., & Larson, J. (1994). Ruminative coping with depressed mood following loss. *Journal of Personality and Social Psychology, 67*, 92–104.

13. Nolen-Hoeksema, S., & Jackson, B. (2001). Mediators of the gender difference in rumination. *Psychology of Women Quarterly, 25*, 37–47.

14. Weissman, M., Bland, R. C., Canino, G. J., Faravelli, C., Greenwald, S., Hwu, H. G., Joyce, P. R., & Yeh, E. K. (1996). Cross-national epidemiology of major depression and bipolar disorder. *Journal of the American Medical Association, 276*, 293–299.

15. Allgood-Merten, B., Lewinsohn, P. M., & Hops, H. (1990). Sex differences in adolescent depression. *Journal of Abnormal Psychology, 99*, 55–63. Also see Blanchard-Fields, F., Sulsky, L., & Robinson-Whelen, S. (1991). Moderating effects of age and context on the relationship between gender, sex role differences, and coping. *Sex Roles, 25*, 645–660. Nolen-Hoeksema, S., Larson, J., & Grayson, C. (1999). Explaining the gender difference in depressive symptoms. *Journal of Personality and Social Psychology, 77*, 1061–1072.

16. Crick, N. R. (1995). Relational aggression: The role of intent attributions, feelings of distress, and provocation type. *Development and Psychopathology, 7*, 313–322. Also see Crick, N. R., & Werner, N. E. (1998). Response decision processes in relational and overt aggression. *Child Development, 69*, 1630–1639.

17. Brown, L. M., & Gilligan, C. (1992). *Meeting at the crossroads: Women's psychology and girls' development.* Cambridge, MA: Harvard University Press.

CHAPTER 4: DRAMA

1. Breath holding spell (n.d.). In *Medline Plus*. Retrieved from http://www.nlm.nih.gov/medlineplus/ency/article/000967.htm. See also Breath holding spells (n.d.). In *Senders Pediatrics*. Retrieved from http://www.senderspediatrics.com/HealthTopics/Health_Topics_A_Z/Behavioral_Emotional_Concerns/Breath_Holding_Spells.page.

2. John, O. P., & Gross, J. J. (2004). Healthy and unhealthy emotion regulation: Personality processes, individual differences, and life-span development. *Journal of Personality, 72*, 1301–1333.

3. Wenzlaff, R. M., & Wegner, D. M. (2000). Thought suppression. *Annual Review of Psychology, 51*, 59–91. And Wenzlaff, R. M., Wegner, D. M., & Roper, D. (1988). Depression and mental control: The resurgence of unwanted negative thoughts. *Journal of Personality and Social Psychology, 55*, 882–892.

4. John, O. P., & Gross, J. J. (2004). Healthy and unhealthy emotion regulation: Personality processes, individual differences, and life-span development. *Journal of Personality, 72*, 1301–1333.

5. Plutchik, R. (2003). *Emotions and life: Perspectives from psychology, biology, and evolution.* Washington, DC: American Psychological Association.

6. Lehrer, J. (2010, February 25). Depression's upside. *New York Times*. Retrieved from http://www.nytimes.com/2010/02/28/magazine/28depression-t.html?pagewanted=all. See also Darwin, C. (2004). *The autobiography of Charles Darwin*. Charleston, SC: BookSurge Classics.

7. Ornstein, R. (1991). *The evolution of consciousness: The origins of the way we think*. New York: Prentice Hall.

8. LeDoux, J. (1996). *The emotional brain.* New York: Simon & Schuster.

9. LeDoux, J. (1996). *The emotional brain.* New York: Simon & Schuster. And Goleman, D. (1995). *Emotional intelligence.* New York: Bantam Books.

10. Goleman, D. (1995). *Emotional intelligence.* New York: Bantam Books.

11. Denham, S., Bassett, H. H., & Wyatt, T. (2008). The socialization of emotional competence. In J. Grusec & P. Hastings (Eds.), *Handbook of socialization* (pp. 614–637). New York: Guilford Press.

12. Calkins, S. D., & Johnson, M. C. (1998). Toddler regulation of distress to frustrating events: Temperamental and maternal correlates. *Infant Behavior and Development, 21*, 379–395.

13. Kang, S. M., & Shaver, P. R. (2004). Individual differences in emotional complexity: Their psychological implications. *Journal of Personality, 72*, 687–726.

14. Tamir, M., John, O. P., Srivastava, S., & Gross, J. J. (2007). Implicit theories of emotion: Affective and social outcomes across a major life transition. *Journal of Personality and Social Psychology, 92*, 731–744.

15. Brown, K. W., & Ryan, R. M. (2003). The benefits of being present: Mindfulness and its role in psychological well-being. *Journal of Personality and Social Psychology, 84*, 822–848.

16. Stegge, H., & Terwogt, M. M. (2007). Awareness and regulation of emotion in typical and atypical development. In J. J. Gross (Ed.), *Handbook of emotion regulation* (pp. 269–286). New York: Guilford Press.

17. These emotion regulation techniques, and others, are well researched by and discussed extensively in Linehan, M. M. (1993a). *Cognitive-behavioral treatment of borderline personality disorder.* New York: Guilford Press. And Linehan, M. M. (1993b). *Skills training manual for treating borderline personality disorder.* New York: Guilford Press.

18. Stegge, H. & Terwogt, M. M. (2007). Awareness and regulation of emotion in typical and atypical development. In J. J. Gross (Ed.), *Handbook of emotion regulation* (pp. 269–286). New York: Guilford Press.

19. LeDoux, J. (1996). *The emotional brain* (p. 175). New York: Simon & Schuster.

20. Goleman, D. (1995). *Emotional intelligence* (p. 21). New York: Bantam Books.

21. Goleman, D. (1995). *Emotional intelligence.* New York: Bantam Books.

22. These techniques follow the "Modal Model" of emotion, which stipulates the effectiveness of modulating emotions through attention, cognitive change, situation selection, situation modification, and response modulation. See Gross, J. J., & Thompson, R. A. (2007). Emotion regulation conceptual foundations. In J. J. Gross (Ed.), *Handbook of emotion regulation* (pp. 3–24). New York: Guilford Press.

23. Barlow, D. H. (1988). *Anxiety and its disorders: The nature and treatment of anxiety and panic* (1st ed.). New York: Guilford Press. And Linehan, M. M. (1993). *Cognitive-behavioral treatment of borderline personality disorder.* New York: Guilford Press.

24. John, O. P., & Gross, J. J. (2004). Healthy and unhealthy emotion regulation: Personality processes, individual differences, and life-span development. *Journal of Personality, 72*, 1301–1333. And, Gross, J. J. (2002). Emotional regulation: Affective, cognitive, and social consequences. *Psychophysiology, 39*, 281–291.

25. Taylor, S. E. (1983). Adjustment to threatening events: A theory of cognitive adaptation. *American Psychologist, 38*, 1161–1173.

26. Leith, K. P., & Baumeister, R. F. (1996). Why do bad moods increase self-defeating behavior? Emotion, risk-taking, and self-regulation. *Journal of Personality and Social Psychology, 71*, 1250–1267.

27. Clark, L. A., & Watson, D. (1991). Tripartite model of anxiety and depression: Psychometric evidence and taxonomic implications. *Journal of Abnormal Psychology, 100*, 316–336. And Linehan, M. M., Bohus, M., & Lynch, T. R. (2007). Dialectical behavior therapy for pervasive emotion dysregulation. In J. J. Gross (Ed.), *Handbook of emotion regulation* (pp. 581–605). New York: Guilford Press.

28. Fredrickson, B. L. (2004). The broaden-and-build theory of positive emotions. *Philosophical Transactions of the Royal Society of London, B, Biological Sciences, 359*, 1367–1378.

29. Gross, E. F. (2009). Logging on, bouncing back: An experimental investigation of online communication following social exclusion. *Developmental Psychology, 45*, 1787–1793.

CHAPTER 5: CHATTERBOX

1. Alexander, B. (2010, June 30). "Sorry guys: Up to 80 percent of women admit faking it." *Sexploration on NBCNews.com*. Retrieved from http://www.msnbc.msn.com/id/38006774/ns/health-sexual_health/t/sorry-guys-percent-women-admit-faking-it. Also see Brewer, G., & Hendrie, C. (2011). Evidence to suggest that copulatory vocalizations in women are not a reflexive consequence of orgasm. *Archives of Sexual Behavior, 40*, 559–564.

2. Kenneally, C. (2007) *The first word: The search for the origins of language* (p. 140). London: Penguin Books.

3. Kenneally, C. (2007). *The first word: The search for the origins of language* (p. 234). London: Penguin Books.

4. Brown, L. M. (2003). *Girlfighting: Betrayal and rejection among girls* (p. 52). New York: New York University Press.

5. Timmers, M., Fischer, A. H., & Manstead, A. S. R. (1998). Gender differences in motives for regulating emotions. *Personality and Social Psychology Bulletin, 24*, 974–985.

6. Timmers, M., Fischer, A. H. & Manstead, A. S. R. (1998). Gender differences in motives for regulating emotions. *Personality and Social Psychology Bulletin, 24*, 974–985.

7. Brown, L. M. (2003). *Girlfighting: Betrayal and rejection among girls.* New York: New York University Press.

8. Brown, L. M., & Gilligan, C. (1992). *Meeting at the crossroads: Women's psychology and girls' development.* Cambridge, MA: Harvard University Press. See also Brown, L. M. (2003). *Girlfighting: Betrayal and rejection among girls.* New York: New York University Press.

9. For more on women and modesty, see Daubman, K., & Sigall, H. (1997). Gender differences in perceptions of how others are affected by self-disclosure of achievement. *Sex Roles, 37*, 73–89, and Brody, L. (1999). *Gender, emotion, and the family.* Cambridge, MA: Harvard University Press.

10. Babcock, J., Waltz, J., Jacobson, N., & Gottman, J. (1993). Power and violence: The relation between communication patterns, power discrepancies, and domestic violence. *Journal of Consulting and Clinical Psychology, 61*, 40–50.

11. Burleson, B. R. (1998). Similarities in social skills, interpersonal attraction, and the development of personal relationships. In J. S. Trent (Ed.), *Communication: Views from the helm for the twenty-first century* (pp. 77–84). Boston: Allyn & Bacon.

12. Dutton, D. G., & Aron, A. P. (1974). Some evidence for heightened sexual attraction under conditions of high anxiety. *Journal of Personality and Social Psychology, 30*, 510–517.

13. Sadalla, E. K., Kenrick, D. T., & Vershure, B. (1987). Dominance and heterosexual attraction. *Journal of Personality and Social Psychology, 52*, 730–738.

14. For a review of the studies described in this section (and others like them), see Guerrero, L. K., Andersen, P. A., & Afifi, W. A. (2011). *Close encounters: Communication in relationships.* Thousand Oaks, CA: Sage Publications.

15. Tolhuizen, J. H. (1989). Communication strategies for intensifying dating relationships: Identification, use, and structure. *Journal of Social and Personal Relationships, 6*, 413–434. See also Owen, W. F. (1987). The verbal expression of love by women and men as a critical communication event in personal relationships. *Women's Studies in Communication, 10*, 15–24.

16. Lee, J. A. (1977) A typology of styles of loving. *Personality and Social Psychology Bulletin, 3*, 173–182.

17. Guerrero, L. K., Andersen, P. A., & Afifi, W. A. (2011). *Close encounters: Communication in relationships.* Thousand Oaks, CA: Sage Publications.

18. For a more nuanced explanation and the possible role of jealousy as a moderating factor, see Miller, S. L., & Maner, J. K. (2009). Sex differences in response to sexual versus emotional infidelity: The moderating role of individual differences. *Personality and Individual Differences, 46*, 287–291.

19. Lennon, R., & Eisenberg, N. (1987). Gender and age differences in empathy and sympathy. In N. Eisenberg & J. Strayer (Eds.), *Empathy and its development* (pp. 195–217). Cambridge, MA: Cambridge University Press.

20. Brody, L. (1999). *Gender, emotion, and the family.* Cambridge, MA: Harvard University Press.

21. Goleman, D. (1995). *Emotional intelligence.* New York: Bantam Books.

22. Etxebarria, I., Ortiz, M. J., Conejero, S., & Pascual, A. (2009). Intensity of habitual guilt in men and women: Differences in interpersonal sensitivity and the tendency towards anxious-aggressive guilt. *Spanish Journal of Psychology, 12*, 540–554.

23. Holley, S. R., Sturm, V. E., & Levenson, R. W. (2010). Exploring the basis for gender differences in the demand-withdraw pattern. *Journal of Homosexuality, 57*, 666–684.

24. Gottman, J. M. (1999). *The seven principles for making marriage work.* New York: Three Rivers Press.

25. Guerrero, L. K., Andersen, P. A., & Afifi, W. A. (2011). *Close encounters: Communication in Relationships.* Thousand Oaks, CA: Sage Publications.

26. Guerrero, L. K., Andersen, P. A., & Afifi, W. A. (2011). *Close encounters: Communication in relationships.* Thousand Oaks, CA: Sage Publications.

27. Falbo, T., & Peplau, L. A. (1980). Power strategies in intimate relationships. *Journal of Personality and Social Psychology, 38*, 618–628.

28. Stern, S. T. (2007). *Instant identity.* New York: Peter Lang.

29. Guerrero, L. K., Andersen, P. A., & Afifi, W. A. (2011). *Close encounters: Communication in relationships.* Thousand Oaks, CA: Sage Publications. For study details, see Giles, H., & Wiemann, J. M. (1987). Language, social comparison, and power. In C. Berger & S. H. Chaffee (Eds.), *Handbook of communication science* (pp. 350–384). Thousand Oaks, CA: Sage Publications.

CHAPTER 6: DRESS UP

1. Dweck, C. S. (2006). *Mindset: The new psychology of success.* New York: Random House. And Dweck, C. S. (2000). *Self-theories: Their role in motivation, personality, and development.* New York: Psychology Press.

2. Dweck, C. S. (2006). *Mindset: The new psychology of success* (p. 13). New York: Random House.

3. Dweck, C. S. (2000). *Self-theories: Their role in motivation, personality, and development.* New York: Psychology Press. Also see Tangney, J. P. (1995). Shame and guilt in interpersonal relationships. In J. P. Tangney & K. W. Fischer (Eds.), *Self-conscious emotions: The psychology of shame, guilt, embarrassment and pride* (pp. 114–139). New York: Guilford Press.

4. Brown, L. M. (2003). *Girlfighting: Betrayal and rejection among girls.* New York: New York University Press.

5. Simmons, R. (2002). *Odd girl out: The hidden culture of aggression in girls* (p. 115). New York: Harcourt.

6. Simmons, R. (2002). *Odd girl out: The hidden culture of aggression in girls.* New York: Harcourt.

7. LeDoux, J. (2002). *The synaptic self.* New York: Penguin Books.

8. LeDoux, J. (2002). *The synaptic self* (p. 40). New York: Penguin Books.

9. Hebb, D. O. (1949). *The organization of behavior: A neuropsychological theory.* New York: Psychology Press.

10. Memory is associative. See Hebb, D. O. (1949). *The organization of behavior: A neuropsychological theory.* New York: Psychology Press.

11. Lomo, T. (1966). Frequency potentiation of excitatory synaptic activity in the dentate area of the hippocampal formation. *Acta Physiologica Scandinavica 68*(277), 128. See also Bliss T., & Lomo, T. (1973). Long-lasting potentiation of synaptic transmission in the dentate area of the anaesthetized rabbit following stimulation of the perforant path. *Journal of Physiology, 232*, 331–356.

12. Kagan, J. (1999). The role of parents in children's psychological development. *Pediatrics, 104*, 164–167.

13. Bavelier, D., Dye, M., & Hauser, P. C. (2006). Do deaf individuals see better? *Trends in Cognitive Sciences, 10*, 512–518.

14. LeDoux, J. (2002). *The synaptic self.* New York: Penguin Books.

15. LeDoux, J. (2002). *The synaptic self* (p. 324). New York: Penguin Books.

16. Eriksson, P. S., Perfilieva, E., Björk-Eriksson, T. Alborn, A. M., Nordborg, C., Peterson, D. A., & Gage, F. H. (1998). Neurogenesis in the adult hippocampus. *Nature Medicine, 4*, 1313–1317. See also LeDoux, J. (2002). *The synaptic self.* New York: Penguin Books.

17. Ford, M. B., & Collins, N. L. (2010). Self-esteem moderates neuroendocrine and psychological responses to interpersonal rejection. *Journal of Personality and Social Psychology, 98*, 405–419.

18. For more on female identity and relationships, see Gilligan, C. (1982). *In a different voice: Psychological theory and women's development.* Cambridge, MA: Harvard University Press. Brown, L. M., & Gilligan, C. (1992). *Meeting at the crossroads: Women's psychology and girls' development.* Cambridge, MA: Harvard University Press. See also Pipher, M. (1994). *Reviving Ophelia: Saving the selves of adolescent girls.* New York: Ballantine.

19. Based on Carol Dweck's *Mindset Theory.* See Dweck, C. S. (2000). *Self-theories: Their role in motivation, personality, and development.* New York: Psychology Press. And Dweck, C. S. (2006). *Mindset: The new psychology of success.* New York: Random House.

CHAPTER 7: KISSING A FROG

1. Lewis, T., Amini, F., & Lannon, R. (2000). *A general theory of love* (p. 99). New York: Random House.

2. Reis, H. T., & Collins, W. A. (2004). Relationships, human behavior, and psychological science. *Current Directions in Psychological Science, 13*, 233–237.

3. Bowlby, J. (1988). *A secure base: Parent-child attachment and healthy human development.* New York: Basic Books. And Ainsworth, M., Blehar, M., Waters, E., & Wall, S. (1979). *Patterns of attachment.* New York: Psychology Press.

4. Lewis, T., Amini, F., & Lannon, R. (2000). *A general theory of love* (p. 63). New York: Random House.

5. Lewis, T., Amini, F., & Lannon, R. (2000). *A general theory of love* (p. 37). New York: Random House.

6. Cozolino, L. (2006). *The neuroscience of human relationships: Attachment and the developing social brain.* New York: W. W. Norton.

7. Cozolino, L. (2006). *The neuroscience of human relationships: Attachment and the developing social brain.* New York: W. W. Norton.

8. Lewis, T., Amini, F., & Lannon, R. (2000). *A general theory of love* (p. 115). New York: Random House.

9. Cozolino, L. (2006). *The neuroscience of human relationships: Attachment and the developing social brain.* New York: W. W. Norton.

10. Lewis, T., Amini, F., & Lannon, R. (2000). *A general theory of love* (p. 141). New York: Random House.

11. Hebb, D. O. (1949). *The organization of behavior: A neuropsychological theory*. New York: Psychology Press.

12. Lewis, T., Amini, F., & Lannon, R. (2000). *A general theory of love* (p. 206). New York: Random House.

13. Lewis, T., Amini, F., & Lannon, R. (2000). *A general theory of love* (p. 120). New York: Random House.

14. Cozolino, L. (2006). *The neuroscience of human relationships: Attachment and the developing social brain*. New York: W. W. Norton.

15. Fletcher, G., & Simpson, J. A. (2000). Ideal standards in close relationships: Their structure and functions. *Directions in Psychological Science, 9*, 102–105.

16. Huston, T. L., Niehuis, S., & Smith, S. E. (2001). The early marital roots of conjugal distress and divorce. *Current Directions in Psychological Science, 10*, 116–119.

17. Dweck, C. S. (2006). *Mindset: The new psychology of success*. New York: Random House.

18. Dweck, C. S. (2000). *Self-theories: Their role in motivation, personality, and development*. New York: Psychology Press. See study, Knee, C. R. (1998). Implicit theories of relationships: Assessment and prediction of romantic relationship initiation, coping, and longevity. *Journal of Personality and Social Psychology, 74*, 360–370.

CHAPTER 8: GOOD GIRLS

1. See table 61 from Centers for Disease Control and Prevention (2010, June 4). *Morbidity and mortality weekly report, 55*(5). Retrieved from http://www.cdc.gov/mmwr/pdf/ss/ss5905.pdf.

2. Centers for Disease Control and Prevention (2010, June 4). *Morbidity and mortality weekly report, 55*(5). Retrieved from http://www.cdc.gov/mmwr/pdf/ss/ss5905.pdf.

3. Guttmacher Institute (2012, February). *Facts on American teens' sources of information about sex*. Retrieved from http://www.guttmacher.org/pubs/FB-Teen-Sex-Ed.html.

4. Tolman, D. L. (2002). *Dilemmas of desire: Teenage girls talk about sexuality*. Cambridge, MA: Harvard University Press.

5. Indiana University Medical Center (2006). *Archives of pediatrics and adolescent medicine*. Retrieved from http://www.msnbc.msn.com/id/14169056/ns/health-sexual_health/t/report-many-teens-dont-use-condoms.

6. Tolman, D. L. (2002). *Dilemmas of desire: Teenage girls talk about sexuality*. Cambridge, MA: Harvard University Press.

7. Blackledge, C. (2003). *The story of V: A natural history of female sexuality* (p. 86). New Brunswick, NJ: Rutgers University Press.

8. Blackledge, C. (2003). *The story of V: A natural history of female sexuality* (p. 87). New Brunswick, NJ: Rutgers University Press.

9. Laumann, E. O., Paik, A., & Rosen, R. C. (1999). Sexual dysfunction in the United States: Prevalence and predictors. *Journal of the American Medical Association, 281*, 537–544.

10. Laumann, E. O., Paik, A., Glasser, D. B., Kang, J. H., Wang, T., Levinson, B., Moreira, E. D., Nicolosi, A., & Gingell, C. (2006). A cross-national study of subjective sexual well-being among older women and men: Findings from the global study of sexual attitudes and behaviors. *Archives of Sexual Behavior, 35*, 145–161.

11. Blackledge, C. (2003) *The story of V: A natural history of female sexuality* (p. 174). New Brunswick, NJ: Rutgers University Press.

12. Diamond, L. M. (2004). Emerging perspectives on distinctions between romantic love and sexual desire. *Current Directions in Psychological Science, 13*, 116–119.

13. Shoda, Y., Mischel, W., & Peake, P. K. (1990). Predicting adolescent cognitive and self-regulatory competencies from preschool delay of gratification: Identifying diagnostic conditions. *Developmental Psychology, 26*, 978–986.

14. Guerrero, L. K., Andersen, P. A., & Afifi, W. A. (2011). *Close encounters: Communication in relationships.* Thousand Oaks, CA: Sage Publications. See study details, Motley, M. T., & Reeder, H. M. (1995). Unwanted escalation of sexual intimacy: Male and female perceptions of connotations and relational consequences of resistance messages. *Communication Monographs, 62*, 355–382.

CHAPTER 9: HOUSEKEEPING

1. Kristof, N. D., & WuDunn, S. (2010). *Half the sky: Turning oppression into opportunity for women worldwide.* New York: Vintage.

2. Rabin, R. (2011, December 14). Nearly 1 in 5 women in U.S. survey say they have been sexually assaulted. *New York Times.* Retrieved from http://www.nytimes.com/2011/12/15/health/nearly-1-in-5-women-in-us-survey-report-sexual-assault.html. Centers for Disease Control and Prevention (2011, November). *The national intimate partner and sexual violence survey (NISVS): 2010 summary report.* Retrieved from http://www.cdc.gov/violenceprevention/nisvs/index.html.

3. Brody, L. (1999). *Gender, emotion, and the family.* Cambridge, MA: Harvard University Press. For a summary of the research, see Glick, P. (1988). Fifty years of family demography: A record of social change. *Journal of Marriage and the Family, 50*, 861–873.

4. Lewin, T. (2011, January 26). Record level of stress found in college freshmen. *New York Times.* Retrieved from http://www.nytimes.com/2011/01/27/education/27colleges.html.

ACKNOWLEDGMENTS

This is written with gratitude to those who have inspired me along the way that led to the writing of this manuscript. The perspective I present in this book is mine, in part, because I was seen in my entirety by both of my parents. Thank you to my mother for our relationship. Her love, warmth, and lesson to believe in the process inspire me daily. Thank you to my editor, T.E.W., for his thoughtful reflection, careful attention, and optimism. To my husband—without his never-ending kindness and absolute belief in me, I would never have completed the first draft. And to our children for bringing unimaginable delight to our lives.

INDEX

About the Author

Jill Weber specializes in the impact of culture on female identity and relationship development. She is a clinical psychologist in private practice in the Washington, D.C., area. She holds a PhD in psychology from American University. She has appeared as a psychology expert in various media outlets including *Nightline*, *Teen Vogue*, *Family Circle*, *Seventeen*, CNN, Associated Press, *U.S. News & World Report*, and the Discovery Channel. Her Web site is www.drjillweber.com.